THE MENOPAUSE HANDBOOK

YOU *CAN* GIVE MENOPAUSE A MISS!

Dr Sandra Cabot

B🌿XTREE

Advice to the reader

The information and procedures contained in this book are based upon the research and the personal and professional experiences of the author. They are not intended as a substitute for consulting with your physician or other health care provider. Before following any dietary or exercise advice contained in this book, it is recommended that you consult your doctor if you suffer from any health problems or special conditions or are in any doubt about its suitability.

Information regarding brand-name products is to the best of the author's knowledge correct at time of going to press.

First published in Great Britain in 1996 by
Boxtree Limited, Broadwall House, 21 Broadwall, London SE1 9PL

Original edition published in Australia in 1991 by
Women's Health Advisory Service, revised 1995

The excerpt on page 212 is from *Always a Woman* by Kaylan Pickford, published by Bantam Books. Reprinted by permission.

1 3 5 7 9 10 8 6 4 2

ISBN: 0 7522 0518 8

Text design and graphics by TJ Graphics
Cartoons by Karen Barbouttis
Cover design by Slatter-Anderson
Front cover image courtesy Ace Photo Agency
Author photo by Laurance Lupton

Printed and bound in Great Britain by The Bath Press, Somerset

A CIP catalogue entry for this book is available from the British Library

CONTENTS

FOREWORD

By Dr Valentine Vargassoff MBBS, FRACP, FRCPA.

Sadly, many women still remain confused, bewildered and out of touch with the tremendous advances in hormonal therapy.

Finally, we have a well-researched, easy-to-read, warm and relatable handbook that puts all the information in a nutshell. Not surprisingly, it has taken a woman doctor, who knows how it feels herself and through her experience with thousands of patients, to awaken women to the tremendous potential of hormone replacement therapy and preventative medicine.

The Menopause Handbook is useful for women of all ages who want to make the time of midlife and beyond a positive and healthy experience. I can thoroughly recommend this book for those wanting to keep pace with the evolution of women during the next decade of the twentieth century.

(Dr Valentine Vargassoff is an Australian physician and pathologist practising in Sydney who specializes in the menopause and breast disorders.)

ACKNOWLEDGEMENTS

I would like to acknowledge the professional and creative assistance of my two editors, Diana Blackwell and Stephanie Lewis, who enabled me to put scientific breakthroughs into everyday language. Without their faith and support this book would not have been so special. I would also like to thank Lydia Sharan for her superb typing skills and her dedication and generosity of spirit, and also Dr Jill McDowell.

PREFACE

The terms 'menopause' and 'change of life' often arouse feelings of fear, dread, uncertainty, and confusion. Yet even though menopause is one of the greatest physical milestones in a woman's life, it does not have to be traumatic or painful.

At around the age of fifty years, the biological clock stops ticking, signalling the loss of fertility and the loss of the sex hormones oestrogen and progesterone. Vitally important questions are raised by the loss of these parts of our identity. Questions such as:

- How will I feel – mentally, physically, and sexually – without sex hormones?
- Will I age more rapidly without oestrogen in my body?
- Will I still be able to function efficiently and compete with younger women in the workplace?
- Will my husband lose interest in me and take a younger lover?
- Will I lose my femininity and look masculine?
- If I have a premature menopause, can I still have a baby?
- Will I get osteoporosis?

Read on and all these questions – and many more – will be answered. This book is your menopause handbook and will serve as a lifeline to guide you through this often awesome and bewildering time of life. It discusses all your options in a simple and clear way, and will leave you fully informed. Most of all, it will take the fear out of menopause and put you back in the driver's seat.

A woman passing through menopause and beyond needs to know about all her options, and is likely to have many unanswered questions about them. For example:

- Do I need to take hormones in the form of hormone replacement therapy?

- Can I use natural hormone replacement therapy instead of the old-fashioned synthetic hormones?
- If one type of hormone replacement therapy doesn't help me, can I take hormones in other forms?
- What is the difference between hormone pills, injections, patches, creams, implants, and suppositories?
- If I don't want hormone replacement therapy, what else can I do to cope with the symptoms of menopause?
- Is there anything I can do to slow down the ageing process?

With the information in this book, you can master the symptoms of menopause and emerge with your vitality, femininity, sexuality and peace of mind intact. Indeed, in many cases the change of life can be a change for the better.

CHAPTER ONE

MENOPAUSE IN A NUTSHELL

My fifty-four-year-old patient had sat for hours on the bus, all the way from an isolated country town called Lightning Ridge, to seek help. She flopped into the chair on the other side of my desk with a desperate and exhausted look in her eyes. She told me that male doctors had no time to listen to her woes and merely threw up their hands, saying that she was 'just getting on in years'. She said that life was cruel for women going through menopause, and that she felt like a sexless, emotionless 'it'. Indeed, she felt as if she had been cheated. She certainly did not want to hear, 'That's life: it's just part of getting older.'

I have heard countless tales like this and – perhaps because I am a woman, too, and not just a doctor – I can empathize with the plight of these frustrated women. But we do not have to suffer the problems of menopause passively. There are real, safe, and simple solutions for today's menopausal woman – solutions to help us recapture our former mental and physical well-being and to slow down the ravages of time on our minds and bodies.

Women are still occasionally told that menopause is part of the Mother Nature's design, and that they should accept it as gracefully as their mothers did. In fact, however, our mothers may have died – as women still die today – from some of the long-term complications of menopause. Fortunately, today's woman has a wide array of choices available – including hormone replacement therapy, counselling, nutritional supplements, dietary modification, and general medical treatment – to help ensure that her passage to midlife and beyond is a fruitful and pleasant voyage.

Figure 1 **Endocrine glands and their hormones**

Follicle stimulating hormone (FSH)
Luteinizing hormone (LH)
both control the ovaries

Growth hormone
regulates growth of body

Prolactin
responsible for milk production

Thyroid hormone
keeps all body systems active

Parathyroid hormone
maintains blood calcium level

Adrenalin
primes body for action

Cortisone
helps manage stress levels

Insulin
maintains blood sugar levels

Oestrogen & Progesterone
control menstruation and maintain pregnancy

(Testosterone controls male sexual characteristics)

Pituitary

Parathyroids

Thyroid

Adrenals

Pancreas

Ovaries
(in men – testes)

WHAT IS A HORMONE?

Before we deal with menopause in depth, it is important to understand what hormones are and how they function in the body. Hormones are body chemicals that carry messages from one part of the body to another. They are made in specialized glands called endocrine glands (see Figure 1) and are circulated in the blood to specific body cells where they make their presence felt.

The thyroid gland manufactures thyroid hormone, the adrenal glands manufacture the adrenal hormones epinephrine (also called adrenaline) and cortisone, and the ovaries produce the sex hormones oestrogen and progesterone. These are just a few of the many hormones required to keep our cells functioning in harmony.

Hormones are concerned with controlling the chemistry of cells. They determine the rate which our cells burn up food and release energy. They also determine whether cells produce milk, hair, secretions, enzymes, or other metabolic products.

Hormones are extremely potent molecules. In some cases, less than a millionth of an ounce of a hormone is sufficient to exert an effect. Individual hormone molecules are far too small to be seen, even under a microscope.

Figure 2 **How hormones affect cells**

Hormones can be likened to chemical 'keys' that turn vitally important metabolic 'locks' in our cells. The turning of these locks stimulates activity within the cells of the brain, intestines, muscles, genital organs, and skin. Indeed, all our cells are influenced to some degree by these amazing hormonal keys. (See Figure 2.)

Without the hormonal keys, the metabolic locks on our cells remain closed and the full potential of our cells is not realized. Imagine a corporation where the employees are unable to communicate with the president and are left to do their own thing. The corporation would lack any unified direction and would be unable to grow. This type of chaos is what would happen in your cells without hormones.

After hormones have completed their tasks, they are either broken down by the cells on which they have acted or are carried to the liver for breakdown. The resulting compounds are then excreted or used again to manufacture new hormone molecules.

CAN HORMONES RUIN YOUR LIFE?

An imbalance in or lack of hormones can shatter your life. Among other things, hormones are vital for making you sexually responsive, passionate, and sensitive, and for sustaining mental drive.

According to consultant gynaecologist John Studd of the Menopause Clinic at King's College Hospital in London, adequate amounts of sex hormones keep women 'out of the orthopaedic wards, the divorce courts and the madhouse'.[1] Before hormone replacement therapy (HRT) became available, a significant percentage of menopausal women suffered a severe midlife crisis that was called, in medical terminology, *involution melancholia*. This old-fashioned term describes the shrinkage of mind and body that can occur without the presence of sex hormones. Some women became so profoundly depressed that they were institutionalized for the rest of their lives.

Hormones control many aspects of human behaviour and emotions, and help to make you a mentally competent, functional person. They are involved in the system of psycho-neuroendocrinology, which is the complex interaction of the mind, the nerves, and the endocrine (hormonal) system. We are only beginning to understand that many mental illnesses, such as manic-depressive illness and schizophrenia, have a chemical basis.

The brain has its own natural 'happy hormones', called endorphins, that act on the pleasure centres in the brain and help us cope with pain and emotional turmoil. If these brain hormones become depleted, you may suffer a deep and gloomy depressive illness. Imbalances of various hormones can create such devastating and insidious signs of malfunction as personality changes, panic attacks, agoraphobia, poor memory, insomnia, frigidity, reduction of sex drive, obesity, blood sugar problems, allergies, and inflammation – and this list is far from exhaustive.

The medical specialization in the treatment of hormonal disorders is called endocrinology. We can now accurately measure the levels of the vast majority of the body's hormones with blood tests, and we are able to replace many of these hormones if the various glands of the endocrine system fail to manufacture them in adequate amounts. This is how the term *hormone replacement therapy* (HRT) came to be.

Hormones – they can make you or break you – make your life heaven or hell, and can be responsible for untold miseries. However, thanks to modern biotechnology, genetic engineering, pharmacology and nutritional medicine, we can now control our hormones. This is truly a powerful medical development, with implications as momentous as the discovery of penicillin.

In this book you will discover the influence of hormones on your mental and emotional state, your ability to succeed, your sexuality and appearance, and the rate at which you age. You will be amazed by the way hormones influence your menstrual cycle, your immune system, and your chances of getting osteoporosis, cancer, and cardiovascular disease.

How Attitudes Have Changed

The attitude of doctors towards menopausal women has changed – slowly – over the last century. In 1850, the most famous gynaecologist of the day, a Frenchman called Colombat, preached to the medical profession that 'all women who have reached this critical period of life should withdraw themselves from the vicissitudes of atmospherical influences, lest they promote plethoric accumulations [congestion with blood] in their regenerative organs, which should henceforth be left in a state of inaction'. He was obviously out of touch with women, to say the least! He was virtually saying that once you're menopausal, you should retire from many of life's passions and pleasures. If men had to experience the discomforts of menopause, we'd probably have had effective treatments for them centuries ago!

Today, many experts regard the postmenopausal phase of a woman's life as a potential 'hormone deficiency disorder', which is a far cry from the negative attitude of doctors such as Colombat. Women's lives are changing, both physically and socially. Our average lifespan has increased from a mere fifty years at the beginning of the 1900s to approximately eighty years today. By the year 2050, it will be ninety-five years or more, and thereafter should continue to increase, according to some predictions. The average woman today spends 40 per cent of her life in a postmenopausal state, so you can understand why the long-term problems of menopause and the postmenopausal years have assumed huge medical, social, and economic significance.

What Causes Menopause?

The word *menopause* means the cessation of menstrual bleeding, which is a sign that oestrogen production has fallen to very low levels. This is due to the inability of the ovaries, the female reproductive organs, to manufacture the sex hormones oestrogen and progesterone. Menopause can thus be called ovarian failure.

WHY DO THE OVARIES FAIL?

This is the million-dollar question. The human female is the only creature known to outlive her sex glands and reproductive capacity. One may well ask, 'Why us? Did Mother Nature go haywire? or are we simply living longer than God intended?'

Even though we may wish it didn't happen, the fact is that our ovaries simply run out of follicles (eggs) at around the age of fifty years. It is the follicles within the ovaries that produce the vast majority of oestrogen and all of the progesterone.

ARE THE OVARIES OF ANY USE AFTER MENOPAUSE?

The ovaries do have an important function after menopause because they can still produce very small quantities of oestrogen and significant amounts of testosterone for a period of approximately twelve years. Thus, the ovaries of a menopausal or postmenopausal woman are certainly not dead, dying, or useless organs. This is why the issue of whether these organs should routinely be removed in menopausal women undergoing hysterectomy remains complex and controversial. If you are faced with this decision, it is wise to obtain several expert opinions.

After menopause, the adrenal glands continue producing – and indeed, may increase their production of – hormones that are then converted into oestrogen in a woman's adipose (fat) tissue. This adrenal gland production of oestrogen may continue for up to twenty years after menopause. The amount of oestrogen produced this way varies, depending on the amount of body fat an individual has and on the health of her adrenal glands. Heavier women, who have more adipose tissue, tend to have higher total levels of oestrogen than thin women. This is probably the reason that heavy women often appear to age more slowly than very thin women. There is no benefit in being underweight as you pass through the menopausal years.

The amount of the hormone testosterone produced by your ovaries is very significant and continues to be so in the postmenopausal years. The ovaries are probably a more potent source of testosterone than the adrenal glands are, and so contribute greatly to sexual desire and enjoyment during the postmenopausal years. In some women, the relatively greater amount of testosterone produced by the postmenopausal ovary may lead to an increase in facial hair, thinning of the hair on the scalp, and shrinkage of the breasts.

Do We Have a Simple Test for Menopause?

The menopausal ovary, being devoid of eggs, is unable to manufacture significant amounts of the female sex hormones. If a blood test is done to measure the levels of oestrogen and progesterone, they will be found to be at low levels. In menopausal and postmenopausal women, blood oestrogen levels (which are measured in the form of oestradiol, the most active form of oestrogen) are generally less than 200 pmol/L. The term pmol/L means picomoles per litre and is a standard laboratory measurement, which is a miniscule amount.

Figure 3 **Low levels of the hormones oestrogen and progesterone**

The function of the ovaries is under the control of the pituitary gland, which is situated at the base of the brain and acts as the master controller for the many hormonal glands in the body. The pituitary gland is very sensitive to the hormonal output of the ovaries, and it begins to react when the ovaries fail to pump oestrogen and progesterone into the bloodstream. The pituitary gland is not at all happy with the failure of the menopausal woman's ovaries. It quickly starts to pump out large amounts of a hormonal messenger called *follicle-stimulating hormone* (FSH), which travels to the flagging ovaries to try to stimulate them back into action (see Figure 3). Alas, the stubborn ovaries have closed up shop for ever and, despite the hormonal pleas and wooing from the pituitary gland, they remain dormant. Meanwhile, the pituitary gland cannot comprehend that the ovaries are unable to respond to its advances and, in a futile attempt to reawaken them, it continues to pump ever-increasing amounts of FSH into the bloodstream. This achieves nothing as far as the ovaries are concerned, but it does provide a useful diagnostic test for your doctor to use to assess whether you are menopausal. Typically, blood FSH levels are quite high if you are menopausal, usually between 40 and 200 milli-international units per millilitre (mIU/ml). This is ten to fifteen times higher than the normal level for premenopausal women.

These blood tests can be very useful if you are suffering from many and vague symptoms for which your doctor can find no obvious cause. Symptoms such as chronic fatigue, rheumatic aches and pains, anxiety, depression, and poor libido may be due to a relative deficiency of oestrogen and progesterone, which is not uncommon in the years leading up to menopause. This time of life is called the premenopause, and though it typically occurs when a woman is in her late forties, it may start at any time after the age of thirty-five. It is often associated with a change in the pattern of the menstrual cycle, with menstrual bleeding becoming erratic – less or more frequent, or heavier or lighter in amount. During the premenopausal years, blood tests to measure the levels of oestrogen, progesterone, and follicle-stimulating hormone may be able to pinpoint a relative deficiency of oestrogen and progesterone. If a deficiency is identified, appropriate hormone replacement therapy can be taken to correct it.

During one of my country trips, a premenopausal woman came up to speak with me after I had given a lecture. She had been complaining of hot flushes, anxiety, panic attacks, headaches, neck aches, and a total loss of libido. She had seen several doctors, who asked her if her menstruation was still regular. As soon as she replied that she menstruated at monthly intervals, their verdict was that she could not possibly be suffering from a deficiency of oestrogen and that her symptoms must be due to stress. She was given prescriptions for sedatives and anti-inflammatory drugs and was told to rest more and cease reading women's magazines. This woman was very angry at her doctors' attitude and was made to feel that she could not cope with the so-called normal phases of life.

A blood test to measure hormonal levels is a simple and relatively non-invasive procedure. It may also be appropriate to try a course of natural hormone replacement therapy for at least three months to see if these premenopausal symptoms can be alleviated. Such treatment can be dramatically effective and often prevents or eliminates the need for sedatives, anti-depressants, painkillers, and anti-inflammatory drugs in premenopausal women.

Some women are told not to worry about their hormones until they stop menstruating completely; once this occurs, they can return to the doctor. But by this stage you may have suffered for years – which in this day and age is no longer necessary – and even your friend will be able to pronounce you menopausal! You won't need a doctor to make the diagnosis.

Many body cells need oestrogen to maintain their normal function. For example, the cells of the vagina, bladder, breasts, skin, bones, arteries, heart, liver, and brain have oestrogen receptors and require oestrogen to stimulate these receptors for normal cellular function. The loss of the three sex hormones –

oestrogen, progesterone, and testosterone – may be associated with an increase in the incidence of heart attacks, high blood pressure and osteoporosis, as well as an increased risk of cancer and abnormalities in the brain's chemistry.

THE FIRST SYMPTOMS OF MENOPAUSE

The signs and symptoms that signal a deficiency of oestrogen can be divided into acute signs (those that occur immediately) and chronic signs (those that occur over the long term). The symptoms that most women notice first are the acute symptoms, including hot flushes, aches and pains, vaginal dryness, bladder problems, dry and ageing skin, sleep difficulties, and a variety of emotional changes.

HOT FLUSHES

Probably the most tell tale sign of all is the onset of hot flushes, or, as they are called in America, hot flashes. You may feel hot and flustered even though everyone else is cool, calm, and collected – and complaining bitterly when you open windows and turn off the heat.

Hot flushes occur because the body's thermostat, situated in the area of the brain known as the hypothalamus, does not function at all well when it is deprived of oestrogen. One minute you may be cold and shivering; the next minute you may feel like an inferno, with an irresistible desire to pull off all your clothes and bedding. One patient of mine told me that her nocturnal hot flushes kept her husband warm all night, so that he no longer needed to turn on the electric blanket. Another patient found her hot flushes extremely embarrassing. They caused her glasses to fog up, and the younger men she worked with thought she was getting hot and excited about them!

Nearly 80 per cent of menopausal women are troubled by hot flushes, and in 70 per cent of this group the flushes will occur, on average, over a period of five years. Hot flushes vary in severity and may be associated with heart palpitations, dizziness, and strange crawling or itching sensations under the skin.

ACHES AND PAINS

Another possible acute symptom of oestrogen deficiency is an increase in bodily aches and pains. For instance, your headaches may become more frequent or severe, your joints may ache, your back and neck may ache, and you may begin to suffer from various rheumatic aches and pains.

VAGINAL DRYNESS

The vaginal tissues are very sensitive to the effect of oestrogen deficiency. More than 50 per cent of menopausal women are troubled by vaginal dryness and failure to achieve adequate lubrication during sexual intercourse. This causes discomfort or pain during sex and, in severe cases, may result in some bleeding from the fragile mucous membrane lining the vagina. Without the strengthening effect of oestrogen, the vagina may become more prone to infection by candida (yeast) and bacteria, which may result in vaginal discharge, itching, and burning.

Over the long term, atrophy (a general shrinkage) of the vagina, the vaginal opening, the vulva (the vaginal lips), and the clitoris may occur. This can have a devastating effect on a woman's sexuality. Fortunately, as we shall see later in the book, there are treatments available that are extremely effective for preventing these changes.

BLADDER PROBLEMS

The tissues of the bladder are also sensitive to oestrogen deficiency. Some menopausal women complain of a frequent and/or urgent desire to pass urine, urge or stress incontinence (a reduced ability to control the passage of urine), a reduced bladder capacity, and an increased susceptibility to cystitis (bladder infection). Needless to say, any of these problems can cause discomfort and/or embarrassment. Fortunately they can be overcome by a combination of pelvic floor exercises, hormone replacement therapy, and/or nutritional measures.

DRY AND AGEING SKIN

Both the superficial and deeper layers of the skin on our faces and bodies are sensitive to oestrogen, as are the collagen fibres that criss-cross in the deeper skin layers. Without oestrogen, the skin becomes thinner and more fragile, more prone to developing discolorations and broken capillaries ('spider veins'), and less capable of retaining moisture. The skin is more prone to dehydration and irritation, and collagen depletion results in a more rapid appearance of wrinkles.

POOR SLEEP

Oestrogen deficiency can adversely affect sleeping patterns, so that difficulty going to sleep or early-morning waking can set in. The problem may be associated with, or made worse by, the occurrence of hot flushes during the night. We know that insomnia is related to oestrogen deficiency because sleep disorders are often helped by hormone replacement therapy, especially if the problem is associated with hot flushes. Studies have shown that taking oestrogen increases the proportion of sleep time spent in the dreaming phase. Many women find that taking oestrogen improves poor memory and decreases irritability. This may be due in part to oestrogen's beneficial effect on sleep.

EMOTIONAL CHANGES

Mental and emotional changes are common at the time of menopause. The most common complaints are depression and anxiety. Personality changes may occur, with rapidly changing moods, irritability, loss of confidence, and panic attacks occurring in women who had none of these problems before menopause. An inability to cope, both mentally and emotionally, is often more poignantly evident in career women who occupy high-profile positions of great responsibility than it is in women who lead less stress-filled lives. Some women say that they feel numb and can no longer muster any passion or *joie de vivre*. If this occurs on a physical level, a woman may experience a total loss of libido and, in extreme cases, she may become completely unresponsive sexually.

AND THEN THERE'S ... YOUR MENTAL ATTITUDE

Your mental attitude is a powerful factor in colouring your personal experience of menopause. Oestrogen deficiency does not affect all women in a negative way. Indeed, some women simply sail through menopause with no emotional changes. Some women find that the cessation of hormonal highs and lows associated with monthly menstrual cycles makes their menopause a time of tranquillity and composure. It is therefore dangerous to stereotype menopausal women, or we could all be brainwashed into having a midlife crisis!

The common emotional changes associated with menopause are not always caused by oestrogen deficiency alone. There may be numerous psychosocial stresses in your life, such as having adolescent children, caring for elderly parents, coping with the altered self-image that comes with ageing, dealing with your husband's midlife crisis, or experiencing 'empty nest syndrome'. All these stresses can take an emotional, mental, and physical toll, especially on the caring, giving type of woman who may find that she is continually supporting others but is receiving no support or

OESTROGEN LEVEL SCORE CHART

The chart below lists acute symptoms that are characteristic of an oestrogen deficiency. It is adapted from a menopause questionnaire devised by Professor Chris Nordin of the Institute of Medical and Veterinary Science at Adelaide University in Adelaide, South Australia.

Rate the severity of each menopausal symptom, as you experience it, and then add up your total score for all the symptoms listed. Use the following scale to rate the severity of your symptoms:

Absent – 0   Mild – 1 point   Moderate – 2 points   Severe – 3 points.

SYMPTOM	SCORE
Depression and/or mood changes	——
Anxiety and/or irritability	——
Feelings of being unloved or unwanted	——
Poor memory and concentration	——
Poor sleeping patterns (insomnia)	——
Fatigue	——
Backache	——
Joint pains, arthritis	——
Muscle pains	——
Increase in facial hair	——
Dry skin and/or sudden development of wrinkles	——
Crawling, itching, and/or burning sensations in the skin	——
Reduction in sexual desire	——
Frequency of or burning sensation with urination	——
Discomfort during sexual intercourse	——
Vaginal dryness	——
Hot flushes and/or excessive sweating	——
Lightheadedness or dizziness	——
Headaches	——
Total score	——

praise in return. If this is true for you, I strongly recommend that you indulge in some well-deserved self-nurturing – take a vacation, arrange for regular massages, practise tai chi, or do something really adventurous!

You may be amazed that the lack of oestrogen can cause such a vast array or diversity of possible symptoms. The reason for this is that receptors for the hormone oestrogen are found on most of the body cells, from the brain to the skin, genital organs, and bones. To assess your own symptoms of oestrogen deficiency, use the Oestrogen Level Score Chart on page 21.

If your total score for all of these symptoms is 15 or more, then it is likely that you are suffering from a deficiency of oestrogen.

If your score is around 30, your body is probably crying out for oestrogen. This can be confirmed or refuted by a simple blood test to check your levels of oestrogen and follicle-stimulating hormone.

We're rapidly approaching the **change of life** when we can look forward to hot flushes, crazy mood swings and chalky bones . . .

. . . while men can look forward to sporty convertibles, gold chains and girlfriends named Leanne.

If you are on hormone replacement therapy, it is an interesting exercise to score your symptoms of oestrogen deficiency both before and after starting HRT. Computing your score every three to four months provides a useful self-check to see whether your hormone replacement therapy is adequate. However, you should not decide to alter your dosage based on the results of this questionnaire without first consulting with your doctor.

I often think back to how it was sixty years ago for women passing through these powerful physiological and emotional changes. In those days, there was little understanding and even less sympathy for the symptoms that women suffered, usually alone and stoically. Thankfully, we no longer live in an era of confusion and ignorance, and women should expect to have their cases heard by sensitive and caring doctors. Once the cause of your symptoms is understood, they can be treated scientifically and effectively. This is a great relief. Women no longer have to feel like helpless victims of the loss of their sex hormones and of the ageing process.

CHAPTER TWO

THE LONG-TERM CONSEQUENCES OF OESTROGEN DEFICIENCY

The life expectancy for women in Western societies today is eighty to eighty-five years. The fastest growing segment of the population in these countries consists of people over fifty-five years of age, and most of these people are women.

When a woman becomes menopausal, she can anticipate another thirty to forty years of life. This means that she will spend around 40 per cent of her lifespan in a postmenopausal state – in other words, without sex hormones in her body. Wow! That sounds fairly dramatic, profound, and perhaps – for the majority of women, who love feeling and acting like women – a little frightening.

The long-term effects of oestrogen deficiency vary among different women, owing to genetic, psychological, and environmental factors. In other words, some women will suffer from effects of oestrogen deprivation, while others will not, and this individuality is obvious to a doctor specializing in this area. Overall, the loss of oestrogen results in a higher risk of osteoporosis, cardiovascular disease, and sexual dysfunction in postmenopausal women.

However, there is much that you and your doctor can do to prevent or offset this higher risk.

VAGINAL ATROPHY

Five years after menopause, most women will have some thinning, dryness, and atrophy (shrinkage) of the vagina, unless they take oestrogen replacement therapy. I have seen quite a few women in their sixties and seventies who have continued to have active and fulfilling sex lives. For the increasing number of women in their seventies and eighties who want to be sexually active, vaginal atrophy is a real concern. However, for many women the biggest problem is not deciding whether to be sexually active, but finding a partner, as on average, men don't live as long as women do.

CARDIOVASCULAR DISEASE

Around 45 per cent of British women will suffer from heart disease or a stroke. Up to the time of menopause, women enjoy a certain amount of protection against cardiovascular disease (diseases of the heart and blood vessels) compared with their male counterparts. Indeed, the incidence of heart attacks in women is only one-third as great as the incidence in men. Unfortunately, after menopause, women begin to lose this relative protection from heart attacks and strokes, so that by the age of seventy-five, a woman's risk of developing these problems is similar to that of man.

MENOPAUSE AND CARDIOVASCULAR RISK

Why are women more prone to cardiovascular disease after menopause? The most important factor appears to be the loss of oestrogen in the body, which results in unfavourable changes in blood cholesterol levels. Not only do overall cholesterol levels tend to rise, but the level of low-density lipoproteins (LDL, or 'bad cholesterol') goes up, while that of high-density lipoproteins (HDL, the so-called 'good cholesterol') goes down. After menopause, this imbalance in cholesterol results in an increase in atherosclerosis (the process of blockage and hardening of the arteries), especially in women who smoke, who are obese, and/or who have sedentary lifestyles.

Early menopause is bad news for your cardiovascular system. Women who lose the function of their ovaries before the age of forty have a greater risk of heart disease than women who go through menopause when they are ten years older. The good news is that large-scale population studies, such as the Framingham Heart Study, have proven that oestrogen replacement can restore a favourable balance in cholesterol levels.

The risk of cardiovascular disease can be reduced by approximately 50 per cent by taking oestrogen at or soon after menopause. A landmark nurses' health study with 48,000 subjects – the first prospective study of women on hormone replacement therapy – found breakthrough results for heart disease.[1] After ten years, it was found that there were half as many cardiovascular deaths and heart attacks among women who took oestrogen after menopause as there were among women who had never used oestrogen.[2] It is important to note, however, that this applies only if natural (not synthetic) oestrogens are used. To put it in a simple way, if you took two large populations of women and gave one group natural oestrogen for twenty-five to thirty years after menopause, but gave no natural oestrogen to the other group, the women who took oestrogen would have half the risk of heart attack as compared with the others. This is because oestrogen reduces total cholesterol levels, increases the proportion of the so-called 'good cholesterol', and prevents cholesterol from being deposited in the walls of the arteries.

The reduction of strokes by hormone replacement therapy appears to be more modest, but it is still significant. A recent study of 23,088 Swedish women showed that postmenopausal oestrogen replacement therapy can reduce the overall risk of stroke by 30 per cent.[3]

We know for sure that oestrogen alone is good for your blood vessels and heart, but we are not sure if taking synthetic progesterone in addition to oestrogen (as is now commonly done) reduces the benefits of oestrogen on your cardiovascular system, particularly if you take oestrogen and progesterone for many years. We are still searching for the ideal progesterone.

Your risk of cardiovascular disease is not determined only by the loss of oestrogen. Other risk factors are equally important – and sometimes more important. These include smoking, high cholesterol levels, a family history of cardiovascular disease, high blood pressure, obesity, lack of exercise, a high-fat diet, and a diet that is deficient in raw foods, fish, and liquids such as water and fresh juices. (See Chapter 6 for ways to minimize these risk factors.)

THE GOOD NEWS ABOUT THE LONG-TERM USE OF HORMONE REPLACEMENT THERAPY

As we continue to live longer and longer, the possible long-term effects of oestrogen deficiency become more and more important. In other words, how might the lack of oestrogen in your body affect you twenty-five to forty years after menopause?

The inaugural scientific meeting of the Australian Menopause Society, held in Brisbane in September 1989, came up with some brain-snapping facts. A study of 8,841 women in a southern California retirement community found that women who had used oestrogen replacement therapy had a significantly reduced risk of death from all causes compared with women who had never taken oestrogen. Much of this was due to a marked reduction in the death rate from heart attacks in women on oestrogen. The lowest death rate was seen in long-term users of oestrogen.[4]

At this meeting, Professor Brian Henderson of the University of Southern California at Los Angeles said that taking natural oestrogen led to a 50 per cent reduction in the risk of heart disease and stroke, giving women an additional 4.2 years of life on average. Another benefit of natural oestrogen cited at the meeting was a lower death rate from some types of cancer. In particular, hormone replacement therapy appears to reduce the risk of cancer of the ovary by up to 40 per cent.[5]

The main benefit of oestrogen in prolonging life comes from its ability to reduce heart disease. This becomes clearer when we look at the total relative risk of death from various causes for women over fifty, summarized in the nurses' study cited on page 26. This study found that there is a 31 per cent overall risk of death from heart disease, a 2.8 per cent risk of death from breast cancer, a 2.8 per cent risk of death following hip fracture, and a 0.7 per cent risk of death from uterine cancer.[6]

So overall, in the long term, we may be better off taking natural oestrogen than not taking it. Still, many women, and many doctors, are reluctant to use adequate doses of oestrogen for sufficient periods of time. Perhaps this is because they still think of HRT as it used to be twenty years ago, when large doses of synthetic oestrogen were taken without the proper balance of progesterone. This resulted in a higher incidence of uterine cancer, blood clots, and high blood pressure. Unfortunately, it also left the impression that all HRT is controversial. This is not so. The natural oestrogens of today are safer so that they cannot realistically be compared to the superhuman doses of synthetic oestrogens that were given years ago. Provided you undergo all the necessary preliminary tests and examinations, the use of natural oestrogen should add years to your life, as well as greatly improve its quality.

OSTEOPOROSIS

Dr Frederick S. Kaplan, a professor of orthopaedic surgery at the University of Pennsylvania, wrote in 1987, 'If hypertension is a silent killer, osteoporosis is a silent thief. It insidiously robs the skeleton of its blanked resources, often for decades, until the bone is weak enough to sustain a spontaneous fracture.'[7]

Osteoporosis has also been called the 'silent epidemic'. It currently afflicts one in every three women in Western society – which is a little depressing, isn't it? But there is some good news. If women take the right precautions early enough, this insidious bone-weakening disease can be prevented. None of these precautions is too hard, and like most things, they're up to us.

Osteoporosis results from the abnormal loss of calcium from the bones, which causes them to weaken and become susceptible to fracture (breakage). It was once thought that osteoporosis was simply a normal part of the ageing process and that it should be accepted gracefully because, after all, it was just a manifestation of Mother Nature's design. We now know this is untrue. Osteoporosis is a disease, and it can be avoided in most cases. Nowadays, no woman should have to suffer its debilitating effects.

Epidemiologists predict that by the year 2050, the world will be full of little old ladies, one-third of them suffering from osteoporosis. I feel that this is unduly pessimistic, as doctors now know how to prevent this disease. I believe that by the year 2050, we will see the good results of preventive medicine reflected in a much lower incidence of osteoporosis than is currently the case.

Today, osteoporosis is very common; by the age of sixty, one in four women living in the Western world develops a significant degree of bone loss. Most women in the early stages of osteoporosis are free of symptoms – so what we're dealing with is indeed a silent epidemic.

By the age of seventy-five, one quarter of all women sustain a fracture of the hip. Nearly one-third of the women who fracture a hip die within six months. Osteoporosis is the twelfth leading cause of death in America. Every year in the United States, some 200,000 hip fractures occur, 85 per cent of them in women. Furthermore, approximately 60,000 of these women die each year. The osteoporosis epidemic increased during the 1970s and 1980s, and appears to be increasing still; indeed, if the tide is not stemmed, we could be looking at half a million hip fractures annually by the year 2000.

By now you are probably shaking in your boots, feeling that it would be easier to avoid death and taxes than osteoporosis. But don't despair. By following a few simple guidelines, you can prevent osteoporosis. The first step is to assess your risk factors.

RISK FACTORS FOR OSTEOPOROSIS

There are a number of definite risk factors that tell if you are likely to develop osteoporosis. Among them are your race, your body type, and lifestyle factors such as diet, exercise, and the use of tobacco and certain medications. (To get an idea of your own risk of developing osteoporosis, see the Osteoporosis Risk Chart on page 31.)

If your total score is under 5 on this scale, you have a low risk of developing osteoporosis.

If your total score is 5 to 8 points, you have a moderate risk of developing osteoporosis.

If your total score is 9 or more points, you have a high risk of developing osteoporosis.

The most accurate way to determine your risk is to have a bone mineral density test done at the time of menopause (see page 39). A bone mineral density (BMD) test is able to determine the density and therefore the strength of your bones. If your bones are dense, then they are more resistant to fracture. A BMD test should be a routine screening test for all menopausal women. It should be considered as essential as a cholesterol test, cervical smear, or mammogram.

Race

The first risk factor for osteoporosis is your racial background. If you are Caucasian or Asian, your chances of developing osteoporosis are higher than they would be if you were black. African-American women tend to achieve greater bone density prior to menopause and experience a slower rate of postmenopausal bone loss.

Body Build

Your body build can be a risk factor. Women with excess weight and those of normal weight are less likely to suffer from

OSTEOPOROSIS RISK CHART

The chart below lists some of the factors that affect your chances of developing osteoporosis. Circle the appropriate scores in the right-hand column and add the numbers up at the bottom to score your own risk.

RISK FACTOR	SCORE
Amenorrhea (lack of menstruation) for:	
6–12 months	1 point
12–24 months	2 points
2–5 years	3 points
5–10 years	4 points
10 years or more (unless you have had a hysterectomy and are receiving adequate hormone replacement therapy, in which case score 0)	
First menstrual period after the age of 17 (late puberty)	1 point
Long-term use of cortisone	5 points
Family history of osteoporosis	3 points
Small, fine-boned frame	2 points
Calcium deficiency during adolescence and/or while nursing a child	2 points
Tobacco use	1 point
Lack of weight-bearing exercise	2 points
Excessive exercise, especially if it leads to amenorrhea	2 points
Caucasian or Asian racial background	1 point
Excessive consumption of protein, salt, alcohol, caffeine, soft drinks	1 point
Overactive thyroid (excess thyroxine)	1 point

Total score   ——

osteoporosis than thin women – so there are some benefits in being a little cuddly, after all! This is because hormones produced by the adrenal glands are converted into oestrogen in the fat, or adipose, tissue. This is a significant source of oestrogen after the ovaries have failed. Being thin, even underweight, may be glamorous for your image, but it is likely to increase your chances of developing osteoporosis. If your bones are very fine – in other words, if your skeletal frame is small – you will be even more likely to develop osteoporosis.

Smoking

Another major risk factor for osteoporosis is smoking. Smoking is bad news for your skeleton because it reduces the production of female hormones by the ovaries, thereby increasing the loss of calcium and other minerals from the bones. This is yet another good reason for women who smoke to kick the habit.

Medications

Taking certain medications may predispose you to osteoporosis. If you swallow large amounts of antacids containing aluminium over a long period of time, this may increase the loss of calcium from your bones. It is preferable to take antacids that are free of aluminium – ask your pharmacist about suitable brands. Avoid using aluminium cooking utensils, as they give you a regular supply of unwanted aluminium. Excessive amounts of aluminium may interfere with calcium metabolism, thereby increasing the risk of osteoporosis.

Cortisone-type drugs also rapidly accelerate the loss of calcium from the bones. If you must take cortisone preparations, you should take them only when absolutely necessary and in the lowest possible dose for the shortest possible time.

Diet

The vital role of diet in the development of osteoporosis was evident to me when I vacationed in Miami Beach in the early 1970s. Miami Beach was then a retirement haven for upper- and middle-class Americans, and one would have expected to see a population of happy, relaxed older women enjoying the good life of the American Dream. On the contrary, I was shocked to see older women who seemed to move slowly and without vitality, many of whom had a 'dowager's hump' – a curvature of the spine creating a rounded hump in the upper back – which is a classic sign of osteoporosis. They seemed older than their years as they plodded along, the curves of their spines forcing them to look at their feet rather than at the sunny skies of Miami.

Ironically, many of these women had brought osteoporosis upon themselves, while living in a land of plenty, because of their long-term consumption of excessive amounts of animal protein, phosphorus (largely found in processed foods), salt, and sugar. A diet like this increases your risk of osteoporosis because it increases the excretion of calcium in the urine and/or disturbs the balance of calcium in the body, so that calcium passes out of the bones and into the blood. We do not need large amounts of animal protein for good health. Many British people consume 100 to 120 grams of protein from animal sources (meat, fish, dairy products) daily, which is more than double what they need. To prevent the loss of calcium, we should consume less than 50 grams of animal protein daily. One 75 gram portion of fish, meat, cheese, or chicken has 21 grams of protein, so you can see how easy it is to consume more than 50 grams.

Periosteum

Cortical bone

Trabecular bone

Figure 4 **The structure of a long bone**

Bones are composed of a dense outer layer, the cortical bone, and a spongier inner layer, the trabecular bone, both contained within a tough, fibrous membrane called the periosteum.

What I was seeing in the early 1970s is now a statistical phenomenon often talked about during conferences on osteoporosis. In Western societies, osteoporosis is becoming a much bigger problem, afflicting ten times as many women as it did in the 1950s and often appearing at a younger age. Experts agree that the reasons must be our lifestyle, diet, and increasing lifespan. Women who drink excessive amounts of alcohol and caffeine are also increasing their risk of osteoporosis, although a modest social intake (for alcohol, no more than four to five alcoholic drinks per week; for caffeine, the equivalent of six to seven cups of coffee per week) does not appear to increase the rate of bone mineral loss.

There are two types of osteoporosis that affect the bones in different ways. Both types of osteoporosis can be influenced by a poor diet.

Bones consist of two primary layers: the *cortical bone*, the dense, compact outer layer, and the *trabecular bone*, the more spongy, porous inner layer (see Figure 4). Type-1 osteoporosis causes a loss of trabecular bone and is mainly due to a lack of sex hormones, specifically oestrogen and androgens. Type-2 osteoporosis causes a loss of cortical bone and is mainly due to deficiencies of calcium and/or vitamin D.

The amount of oestrogen produced by your body is affected by the amount of calories you consume. If you are a chronic dieter and consume a very low calorie diet, and especially if your menstrual periods are infrequent and light, you may suffer from a premature oestrogen deficiency, which can lead to type-1 osteoporosis.

You are more likely to suffer from type-2 osteoporosis if your diet is specifically lacking in calcium and/or vitamin D. The recommended daily allowances (RDAs) for calcium are 800 milligrams for premenopausal women and 1,000 milligrams for menopausal and postmenopausal women. It is alarming to learn that *three-quarters of all women fail to consume these RDAs*. This sets the stage for the development of type-2 osteoporosis. By eating plenty of calcium-rich foods, you can ensure that you get at least the RDA of calcium each day. (See Chapter 6 for information about food sources of calcium.)

Your intake of calcium during adolescence and when you are in your twenties is crucial in determining your peak bone mass (the ultimate mass that your bones achieve). Today, many adolescent girls are reducing their peak bone mass by stringent dieting and excessive exercise. This will increase their risk of developing osteoporosis later in life.

The ratio of calcium to other minerals in the diet is also important. The ratio of calcium to phosphorus, for example, should be 2:1. Yet the modern-day Western diet contains so much phosphorus that the balance has tipped in favour of phosphorus by 4:1. This excess of phosphorus can speed up loss of calcium from the bone. You should aim to reduce the amount of high-phosphorus foods in your diet by avoiding products whose labels include ingredients such as phosphoric acid, sodium and potassium phosphate, polyphosphate, and pyrophosphate. Generally, phosphorus and its derivatives are found in processed or canned meats; processed cheeses; any processed foods that are laden with artificial preservatives, flavourings, and colourings; packaged cookies and pastries; fizzy soft drinks; and packaged breads and cereals. By now you are probably wondering where your nearest health food store is, as many of the products found at your local supermarket or convenience store are loaded with phosphate additives.

The mineral magnesium is important in helping your body to utilize calcium. If you increase your intake of calcium, you should raise your intake of magnesium as well. The ideal calcium to magnesium ratio is 2:1; therefore, if you consume 1,000 milligrams of calcium a day, you need 500 milligrams of magnesium daily. If you take these minerals in supplement form, it is possible to obtain tablets containing both calcium and magnesium in the correct ratio of 2:1.

The antioxidant vitamins C and E are important as well. They are necessary for the manufacture and maintenance of the tough fibrous collagen in our bodies. Collagen gives our bones flexibility, making them less brittle and more resilient in the face of sudden stresses.

A deficiency of vitamin D may also predispose you to developing osteoporosis. Vitamin D deficiency has been found in 30 per cent of postmenopausal women with bone deterioration.[8] Unlike other vitamins, vitamin D is actually a hormone that is synthesized in your skin when it is exposed to direct sunlight. However, many women now choose to avoid the sun as much as possible because of its ageing effects on the skin. You can also obtain vitamin D from liver, especially fish liver, fatty fish such as halibut, mackerel and salmon, butter, eggs, and vitamin-D-enriched milk. Women who are likely to suffer a vitamin D deficiency include those with food-absorption or digestive problems and intolerances to any dietary fat, as well as those who get no exposure to sunlight. If any of these applies to you, you should consult your doctor for a blood test to measure your level of vitamin D and determine whether you need vitamin D supplements, and, if so, at what dosage. Generally speaking, a daily supplement of 400 international units of vitamin D is adequate and safe.

Other nutrients that help calcium keep your bones strong and healthy are boron, vitamin K, copper, zinc, manganese, and silica. A good multiple vitamin and mineral table should contain all of these nutrients.

Exercise

Women who do not get regular weight-bearing exercise are at far greater risk of developing osteoporosis than those who do. Weight-bearing exercise is not the same thing as weight-lifting. It is any type of exercise that involves movement in the upright position, so that body weight is being transmitted through the spine, pelvis, and legs to the ground – in other words, the force of gravity acts vertically downwards on the skeleton. Ideally, this exercise should involve muscular contraction. Examples of suitable weight-bearing exercise include thirty minutes daily of walking, jogging, aerobics, or yoga. It is best to choose a form of exercise that you can adopt as a lifestyle. However, you should be aware that too much exercise can reduce body fat excessively, causing oestrogen levels to drop. In extreme cases, menstruation may cease. If this happens, it reflects a dangerously low oestrogen level – and increases your risk of developing osteoporosis. Moderation in exercise is the key .

Heredity

Genetic factors are important in determining how dense your bones will become. Consider yourself to be at a higher than average risk if your mother, grandmother, or sister has developed osteoporosis. Fortunately, you can help to offset this increased risk by adopting a healthy lifestyle and eating a high-calcium diet.

Menopause – THE Most Important Risk Factor

The loss of the hormone oestrogen at the time of menopause is the major cause of osteoporosis. If women did not go through menopause, their incidence of osteoporosis would be closer to that of men – that is, it would be approximately twenty times lower. The earlier the menopause, the longer a woman spends in the postmenopausal state, and the greater her chances for developing osteoporosis. Women who experience premature menopause are at particular risk. But the women most at risk are those who have had their ovaries surgically removed, especially if this is done before they reach the age of forty-five, and who have never received adequate hormone replacement therapy.

If you have a combination of several risk factors, your chances of developing osteoporosis are multiplied. You should therefore do everything possible to remove these risks and decrease your chances of developing the disease. For example, if you are thin, eat a poor diet, smoke cigarettes, drink alcohol excessively, and reach menopause before the age of forty-five, you are a prime candidate for developing osteoporosis. Fortunately many, if not most, of these risk factors are things that you can control.

THE SIGNS OF OSTEOPOROSIS

Unfortunately, in many cases, the first sign of osteoporosis is the fracture of a bone, particularly in the wrist, hip, or spine, after minimal damage or trauma. To avoid this painful outcome, you should be aware of the signs that may indicate the earlier stages:

- A gradual reduction in height. If your dresses and trousers seem to be getting longer, that may be a warning sign.
- A stooping of the spine and rounding of the shoulders. This happens when the normally square-shaped spinal vertebrae gradually collapse into triangular wedges. If this is allowed to continue, you may develop a hump on your spine, below the neck, that is rather disparagingly called a 'dowager's hump'.
- General aches and pains in the bones may signal early osteoporosis, so remember, all that aches is not necessarily arthritis. Be wary of accepting anti-inflammatory arthritic medication or painkillers without first having tests done for osteoporosis.
- If the texture of your skin changes, rapidly losing its thickness and suppleness at the time of menopause, then it is more likely that collagen loss is occurring in the bones. It is the loss of collagen fibres in the dermal layer of the skin that causes sudden wrinkling and loss of texture. Brittle nails and deterioration of the teeth may also be a clue. According to experts at King's College in London, the development of osteoporosis is due partly to a loss of collagen in the bones, which causes them to become excessively brittle. The loss of collagen in the bones is often mirrored by a loss of collagen in the skin.

IS THERE A RELIABLE TEST FOR OSTEOPOROSIS?

Doctors have a test called a bone mineral density (BMD) test that can accurately predict your chances of developing osteoporosis. The BMD test measures the concentration of minerals in your bones to determine how strong and resistant to fracture the bones are.

Ideally, all women should have a BMD test when they pass through menopause, not several years later, as bone mineral loss can be rapid in the first five years after menopause. Ask your doctor for a referral to a medical facility experienced in administering the BMD test. Ideally, such a facility should be equipped with the latest lunar DPX-L bone densitometer machines, which utilize dual energy X-ray absorptiometry (DEXA) technology. Measurements of bone density should be made in the spine and hips. By the way, ordinary X-rays are not an accurate test for osteoporosis.

The BMD test takes fifteen to twenty minutes to perform and does not involve any injections, drugs, or discomfort. It is accurate to within one half of 1 per cent and emits less radiation than a dentist's X-ray. It really is an ideal test that your doctor can use to monitor your bone density at regular twelve- to twenty-four-month intervals over many years and give you peace of mind.

Figure 5 illustrates the acceleration of bone loss that often occurs when a woman passes into the oestrogen deficiency zone of menopause. The dotted line represents the bone fracture threshold, which is the point at which bone mineral density becomes so low that a bone may fracture under the slightest stress. In the unfortunate women whose bones reach this threshold, the fracture of a hip may occur simply as a result of jumping out of bed and putting all the weight on one hip; a vertebral compression fracture in the spine can be caused by sitting in a car travelling over a rough road. Indeed, if your bone density crosses the fracture threshold, you become a virtual 'china doll'.

In Figure 5 you can see that the time zone around menopause, represented by the shaded column, is a crucial time corridor where

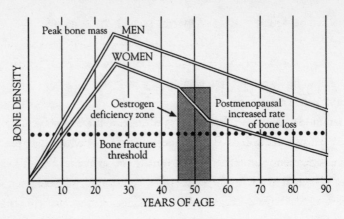

Figure 5 **The increased risk of bone fracture associated with menopause**

The diagram above shows the change in average bone mass for women, by age; the dotted line represents the point at which the bone density is so low that a fracture may occur with only the slightest stress. Notice that bone loss is most rapid between 45 and 55 years – the period around menopause.

the loss of bone mass can be greatly accelerated. Indeed, because of the loss of oestrogen during this time, a rapid bone-loser can lose a large amount of her total bone mass. More than 50 per cent of the total amount of bone that is lost in the postmenopausal years is usually lost in the first seven to ten years after menopause. A new blood test to identify your risk of osteoporosis should become available within the next few years. It is based on the fact that researchers have identified a gene that determines bone strength or density.

PREVENTING OSTEOPOROSIS

The current epidemic of osteoporosis in women aged sixty and above reflects the fact that ten years ago there was no accurate test to discover the very early stages of this disease. Consequently, these women came for medical attention only when they had developed bone fractures or humping of the spine. And unfortunately, at this advanced stage it is difficult to put back the calcium that has leached out of the bones. But the good news is that we can prevent the loss of calcium from the bones if treatment is begun early, at the time of menopause – not ten years later.

Hormone Replacement Therapy

Hormone replacement therapy is an effective method of preventing osteoporosis. Ideally, HRT should begin when the deficiency of sex hormones first becomes apparent – usually at the time of menopause or, in some women, in the premenopausal years. Many studies have shown HRT to be effective treatment for the maintenance of bone size and strength and the prevention of bone fractures. HRT must be taken for fifteen to twenty years to prevent osteoporosis effectively.

After three years of treatment, women who receive oestrogen therapy have about 10 per cent more bone than those not on HRT. Figure 6 shows the effect of oestrogen therapy in slowing the rate of bone loss. One in three women is what we call a 'fast bone-loser'. In such women, oestrogen replacement is able to slow the rate of bone loss so that the fracture threshold is never crossed.

HRT is a powerful tool against osteoporosis because it not only reduces the loss of minerals from the bone, but slows the loss of collagen from the skeleton as well. It also slows the loss of collagen from the deeper layers of the skin, and it is thought that this effect slows the rate of ageing of the skin. It seems that HRT is not only good for your inner layers but also for your outer layer!

Osteoporosis can cause the bony vertebrae of the spine to become weak and spongy, and their once-rectangular solid forms to be crushed into triangular wedges. These are called compression fractures (see Figure 7). Compression fractures cause a loss of height, a protruding abdomen, and a curved posture, with compression of the spinal nerves that causes sharp shooting pains in the spine and limbs. Currently, one in four Australian women over the age of sixty-five has one or more spinal compression fractures, and one estimate suggests that about 60% of elderly women in the UK will experience wedging of bones in the spine.

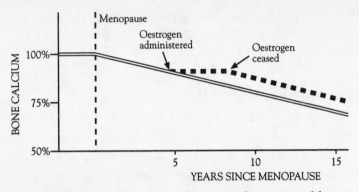

Figure 6 **The effect of oestrogen therapy on bone mineral loss**

In this diagram, the solid line shows the rate at which the bones lose calcium in the years after menopause; the dotted line shows the effect of oestrogen therapy. It demonstrates that oestrogen therapy can virtually halt the loss of calcium from the bones, although when oestrogen is discontinued, calcium loss resumes.

A loss of bone mass also commonly occurs in the hips, and without preventive treatment, 50 per cent of postmenopausal women are at risk of a hip fracture by the age of seventy-five. Taking oestrogen replacement therapy for fifteen years after menopause postpones the age of high fracture risk to ninety years. Currently, the British Medical Association's estimate of average healthy lifespan is eighty-five years, so HRT in effect enables the majority of women to escape fractures. Women who use oestrogen therapy have a 60 per cent lower risk of osteoporotic fractures than women who do not.[9] As women continue to live longer, they may need to take HRT for longer periods; the ideal solution would be to reprogramme the ovaries to pump out oestrogen indefinitely.

In addition to oestrogen, some progestogens have worthwhile ability in reducing bone loss. This provides another reason for combining oestrogens and progestogens in HRT prescriptions.

Calcium Supplementation
Calcium plays a role in building up your peak bone mass and reducing the bone loss associated with ageing and menopause. Bone fracture rates in the elderly are reduced when adequate

Figure 7 Compression of the spinal vertabrae

Compression fractures occur when the normally rectangular vertebrae, weakened by osteoporosis, are crushed into triangular wedges, causing a reduction in height and changes in posture.

calcium intake is maintained. Professor Chris Nordin of Adelaide University in South Australia is a brilliant authority on calcium metabolism. He recommends that you take 500 milligrams of calcium daily if you consume dairy products regularly, and 1,000 milligrams daily if you do not. Table 9, in Chapter 6, will enable you to make sure that your diet and calcium supplements provide you with at least 1,000 milligrams of calcium daily. It has been found that fewer than 40 per cent of menopausal women have an adequate daily intake of calcium.

Calcium supplements are best taken last thing at night, just before you go to bed, because it is during sleep and when your stomach is empty that blood calcium levels fall. To replace it, parathyroid hormone dissolves precious calcium from your bones. By taking calcium before sleep, you can prevent this.

Anabolic Steroids

Anabolic steroids are male hormones (natural and synthetic) that are well known for their infamous role in competitive sports, yet few people know that they are often used to help women with established osteoporosis. The rationale for their use is that menopausal women with high blood levels of testosterone lose bone more slowly than women with lower testosterone levels. The role that anabolic steroids play is not clear, but they have been shown to help prevent bone loss and may even bring about some degree of bone gain in cases of established osteoporosis.

Anabolic steroid tablets and injections may be very useful for women with osteoporosis who are unable to take oestrogen. You should be aware, however, that these drugs can cause oily skin, pimples, fluid retention, and weight gain, as well as an increase in facial hair, deepening of the voice, and loss of libido. As a result, some women who try them discontinue use of them. On the other hand, many women find that these drugs reduce musculo-skeletal pains and greatly increase vitality.

Regular Daily Exercise

Exercise is a vitally important strategy for preventing osteoporosis. As discussed earlier in this chapter, the right kind of activity is a weight-bearing exercise such as walking, jogging, aerobics, or yoga, done for thirty to forty minutes every day. You should avoid over-exercising, however (see page 37).

TREATMENTS FOR OSTEOPOROSIS

Unfortunately, there is no cure for osteoporosis. There are, however, a number of medical treatments available that show some promise for treating the disease.

Etidronate

This drug reduces the resorption (loss) of bone and is most useful for women with severe osteoporosis and those unable to take oestrogen. It can restore the strength of demineralized bone and reduces the frequency of spinal fractures.[10] Etidronate is sold by prescription under the brand name Didronel. It is also used as a treatment for Paget's disease (another bone disease that chiefly afflicts the elderly) and certain metabolic disorders. If you think you might be interested in trying etidronate, I suggest you consult a bone specialist, preferably one who has a particular interest in osteoporosis, who is experienced in using this drug and may be comfortable treating you with it. Etidronate is a biphosphonate drug and newer types of these drugs with fewer side-effects are becoming available.

Calcitonin

Calcitonin is a natural hormone that is extracted from salmon or eels. It delays bone loss both during and after menopause, even in older women with established osteoporosis. It is sold under the brand names Calsynar and Miacalcic.

At present, calcitonin is expensive and must be taken by daily injection (a home injection kit is available). A nasal spray form is currently under research, and hopefully will be available soon. This would make it much easier to use, and it could become a very useful alternative for the prevention and treatment of osteoporosis, especially for many women who are unable to take oestrogen replacement therapy.

Calcitriol

Calcitriol (vitamin D3) is the active form of natural vitamin D. It is sold under the brand name Rocaltrol. A large scientific trial in women with postmenopausal osteoporosis showed that over a three-year period, calcitriol reduced the incidence of new spinal fractures by 70 per cent and that of other bone fractures by 50 per cent.[11] Although this is encouraging, other studies have found it has less benefit for the bones in the limbs, while confirming that it strengthens the spine. If you take calcitriol, you must not also take calcium supplements unless you check with your doctor first.

All of these treatments are encouraging, but the fact is that modern medicine still does not have the ability to reverse severe established osteoporosis. What doctors can do extremely well is to prevent osteoporosis by the use of treatment in the premenopausal, menopausal, and postmenopausal years. Do not be lulled into a false sense of security; start taking precautions in the premenopausal years, and you won't be robbed by the silent thief in the years ahead.

Preventing osteoporosis is important not only for our individual well-being, but also for the sake of society as a whole. The percentage of older persons in our population is increasing, and while today's affluent society has the resources to care for the health of these people, this may not always be so. Epidemiologists estimate that by the year 2025, the percentage of persons under fifteen years of age will have gone from approximately 35 per cent (in 1901) to approximately 19 per cent, while the percentage of persons over sixty-four years of age will have increased from approximately 4 per cent to approximately 16 per cent. The smaller number of younger persons will find it increasingly difficult to support the health of the larger number of older persons, both financially and socially. To avoid the higher cost to society of providing health care for our ageing population, we must use the tools of preventive medicine while we are in midlife.

Moreover, women generally outlive men, and a large number of widows will spend around a decade without their partners. If they cannot maintain mental, emotional, and physical health, they may be forced into nursing homes and institutions, where care is expensive and their health may deteriorate further.

I do not want to sound like a prophet of doom, however. Rather, I want to help you realize that you are likely to have a better menopause and postmenopause if you take active responsibility for your own mental and physical health. This means ensuring that your doctor assesses your risk of cardiovascular disease, osteoporosis, cancer, and degenerative diseases at the time of your menopause. If such problems are found at this early stage, they can be corrected and further deterioration prevented.

We know that if hormone replacement therapy is given for ten to fifteen years after menopause, we achieve a large reduction in the incidence of heart attacks, stroke, and bone fractures. Theoretically, such reductions in these common diseases that afflict older women should become more evident as hormone replacement therapy is continued beyond the age of sixty-five.

Looking at these statistics, you may be convinced that every menopausal woman should have HRT. However, this is not necessarily the case. Each woman is unique. For example, some menopausal women have no troublesome symptoms and are not at risk of cardiovascular disease or osteoporosis, as determined by a bone mineral density (BMD) test and total physical examination. Such low-risk women have no medical need for HRT. However, they may still decide to take HRT for personal reasons, such as the desire to maintain a more youthful appearance or a more fulfilling sex life.

Whether you decide to take HRT or not, it is wise to begin a lifestyle and nutrition programme for preventive health care. Strategies like getting regular exercise and increasing your intake of low-fat, high-calcium, and high-fibre foods, as well as raw fruits and vegetables, are probably more important than the decision to take hormone replacement therapy alone. Full details on diet, nutritional supplements, and exercise for midlife and beyond will be discussed in Chapters 6 and 7.

I believe that we can become what we visualize ourselves to be. Give yourself positive affirmations; tell yourself that you will be strong, energetic, and mentally switched-on as you age, and work towards these goals every day in a practical way. Don't let anyone convince you that your health must decline with age. I have witnessed thousands of women who have improved with age, and who have actually started to look and feel younger once they began using the miraculous healing tools of modern and naturopathic medicine together with a healthy lifestyle.

CHAPTER THREE

YOUR VISITS TO THE DOCTOR

I recommend that all women visit their doctors annually for a complete physical examination. In this way, problems can be detected early, and we all know that prevention is better than cure. It is essential that you develop a good rapport with your doctor and feel comfortable about expressing your deepest concerns. Don't worry if it takes a little searching to find a doctor you feel at ease with.

An annual check-up is important even if you do not want hormone replacement therapy or other prescription treatments. If you are more interested in natural health care alternatives, you may want to find a doctor who specializes in, or at least is knowledgeable, about these areas. Some women prefer to visit both a doctor and a natural therapist, so that they can have the best of both worlds. This is a good idea, although unfortunately it may be a little too expensive for some.

Women who do not experience unpleasant symptoms at menopause may be reluctant to consult a doctor, or may think there is no reason to, because they have no need or desire to have any 'treatment'. It should be emphasized that menopause is not a disease, and it is important not to medicalize it by taking an overly interventionist approach. However, the risk of certain serious diseases rises rather sharply at this time of life, so regular physical examinations become more important than ever before for the maintenance of your good health.

Whatever your situation, a good doctor should take your individual perspective and needs into account. In addition, because the changes that menopause produces in your body are gradual, both you and your doctor should be aware that your needs and feelings may change over time. There is no need to rush into any treatment or to feel pressured by a doctor; the goal is to stay in tune with your body and work with your doctor to optimize your health.

This chapter will give you a good idea of what to expect at those all-important medical check-ups.

YOUR FIRST VISIT

I suggest you consult a gynaecologist or a doctor who has a special interest in women's health when you first experience premenopausal symptoms. If you are one of those lucky women who experiences no premenopausal symptoms, you should visit a doctor once you realize that menopause is taking or has taken place. Your first visit should be around thirty to forty minutes long, thus allowing time for a full history and physical examination. I am afraid to say that the most attentive level of care you will get is likely to be through seeing a doctor privately. The restrictions of time and money on doctors seeing patients on a National Health Service basis with the way the system currently operates means, for instance, that it is unlikely that an NHS doctor or gynaecologist will be able to see you for as long as thirty to forty minutes. But try to make sure he or she answers all your questions and concerns, and bear in mind the points I have outlined below.

YOUR HISTORY

Before deciding what medical treatment, if any, is appropriate for you, your doctor must take a medical history and perform a full physical check-up and a battery of tests. At the time of menopause, your ovaries, adrenal glands, and adipose (fat) tissue may still produce enough sex hormones to keep you feeling well. In the ten years after menopause, your levels of sex hormones will gradually decline, and at some point you may feel a desire to try hormone replacement therapy. Your doctor will then want to know if there are any risk factors in your family history that could influence the decision to begin HRT. For instance, if you have a strong family history of breast cancer – if close relatives have had the disease, and especially if it was diagnosed before menopause – your doctor would be more conservative about giving you oestrogen replacement. Conversely, if you have a family history of osteoporosis or cardiovascular disease, your doctor would probably be more likely to advise you to take oestrogen replacement on a long-term basis, as this would reduce your chances of following in your relatives' footsteps.

Particular attention should be paid to your menstrual pattern. If you have had irregular bleeding, or any bleeding after regular menstruation has stopped for twelve months, you should have a curettage of the uterus or a hysteroscopy performed before beginning HRT. Curettage of the uterus is a procedure in which the lining of the uterus is scraped away so that it can be examined under a microscope for the presence of abnormal cells. Hysteroscopy is a relatively new procedure in which the doctor passes a flexible telescope through the opening of the cervix into the inner cavity of the uterus to view the uterine lining; if abnormal tissue is seen, this can then be biopsied (sampled). Both of these are usually outpatient (same-day) procedures performed under general anaesthetic. They are done to rule out the possibility that bleeding is being caused by uterine or cervical cancer. If either of these conditions is discovered, urgent treatment, usually surgery, will be required. If cancer is ruled out as a cause of irregular bleeding, we can say that the bleeding is due to hormonal changes.

If you are interested in taking HRT, a previous history of gynaecological cancer is very significant. If you have had successful treatment of a previous cancer of the ovaries or cervix, then HRT should not be a problem. However, if you have had endometrial cancer (a cancer of the inner lining of the uterus) – even if the cancer was treated successfully – taking oestrogen could theoretically stimulate a recurrence. Check with the gynaecologist and/or the oncologist (cancer specialist) who treated your cancer before making a decision regarding HRT.

Your past history of other medical problems is also worth

scrutinizing. A woman's risk of developing cardiovascular disease rises significantly at menopause, so detection and treatment of high blood pressure, heart disease, or blood clots, for example, becomes important at this time. In addition, if you have had any of these problems, special care is needed in making a decision about HRT, specifically in deciding the type of HRT that is best for you. Your doctor will also want to know about your lifestyle and daily habits, as well as your expectations and needs concerning your sex life. Ideally, before starting HRT, if you smoke, you should stop; if you lead a sedentary life, you should begin to exercise regularly; and if you are overweight, you should slim down.

Your doctor will also quiz you about your menopausal symptoms, such as hot flushes, to assess your level of oestrogen deficiency. Why not make it easier for your doctor by taking along your completed oestrogen deficiency score chart? (See page 21.)

If you are enjoying an active and fulfilling sex life, you can optimistically anticipate that it can continue through menopause. HRT in particular can be helpful in ensuring a lasting quality to this pleasure. It definitely helps with vaginal and vulval lubrication and the ability to achieve a satisfying orgasm, as well as preventing shrinkage of the breasts, uterus, vagina, and clitoris. Most women want to remain sexually active way beyond menopause.

Finally, your contraceptive needs should be discussed, because until your menstrual cycles stop completely, you may still be ovulating, at least occasionally. This means that there is theoretically still a slight risk of pregnancy. And even if you decide to take HRT, that does not guarantee 100 per cent protection against pregnancy, as hormone replacement is not as effective in suppressing ovulation as the oral contraceptive pill. If you are premenopausal or in the early stages of menopause, when there is still a change of ovulation, you have a number of contraceptive choices.

If you prefer oral contraceptives, you can take the so-called 'mini-pill' (an oral contraceptive containing progesterone only, rather than a combination of oestrogen and progesterone), along with natural oestrogen, until it is certain that menopause has arrived. If you are perimenopausal (in the years leading up to, during, and just after the final menstruation, aged approximately forty-five to fifty-five) and are not taking HRT, you can use either the mini-pill alone or a low-dose combination contraceptive pill. The mini-pill will offer you a greater than 95 per cent protection against pregnancy, and in many cases much better if ovulation is infrequent. A low-dose combination contraceptive pill will give you greater than 99 per cent protection. If you are a smoker or have high blood pressure, it is safer to avoid all contraceptive pills containing oestrogen, although the mini-pill, which contains progesterone only, can be used safely. Alternatively, physical methods of contraception – such as the diaphragm, intrauterine device (IUD), or condoms – can be used until menopause has definitely arrived.

Generally, doctors recommend that you use some form of contraception until you have had no menstrual periods for a year. After that, you should be able to relax and stop worrying about pregnancy. It is extremely unlikely you would conceive after more than a year without a menstrual period. Also, if you have an elevated blood level of follicle-stimulating hormone (over 30 milli-international units per millilitre; see page 15), that would indicate you are menopausal and therefore beyond your fertile stage.

THE VITAL PHYSICAL EXAMINATION

The physical portion of the examination should take at least ten to fifteen minutes, and you'll be required to get into your birthday suit for the occasion. Your doctor will check your weight, pulse, and blood pressure; listen to your heart; and inspect your blood vessels, especially the veins in your legs. The thyroid gland, that soft, fleshy mound in the front of your Adam's apple, will be pressed, and your doctor should palpate (examine with his or her hands) your neck and armpits for any lumps or swelling. Your breasts should be thoroughly examined for any tenderness, lumpiness, or thickening. The skin and nipples of the breast should also be inspected. Then your abdomen will be checked.

Figure 8 **The pelvic examination**

Finally, the doctor will do a pelvic examination (see Figure 8). The vagina and vulva should be checked for signs of oestrogen deficiency or disease processes. The mucous membrane lining the vulva and vaginal wall will be checked, and an instrument called a speculum will be gently inserted to open up the vagina to expose the cervix. This allows a cervical smear to be taken (see Figure 9). This is a procedure in which the doctor scrapes cells from the cervix, using a spatula or a small brush. These cervical cells are then examined under a microscope for signs of changes that may signal developing cancer.

In a woman with an oestrogen deficiency, the vaginal secretions are scanty and alkaline (non-acidic), and the mucous membrane lining the vulva and vagina may be thin and fragile. Understandably, in such cases the taking of a smear may be uncomfortable. It may be necessary to use a vaginal oestrogen cream for one month to restore the vaginal tissues to normal so that a smear and pelvic examination can be done comfortably.

You will be asked to cough or bear down while your doctor views the vaginal opening. This is done to reveal any tendency to prolapse of the uterus, bladder, and/or vagina, a situation that occurs when the ligaments and muscles supporting these organs weaken, causing them to fall downward and protrude through the vaginal opening. Next comes what I affectionately call the 'squeeze test', as the doctor palpates with two hands your uterus, ovaries, and surrounding pelvic organs. This is a vital part of your check-up, as the only early evidence of cancer of the ovary is a swelling or lump in the pelvis. Try to relax and breathe deeply during this procedure. It will make the pelvic examination more comfortable – and far more accurate. Making sure you have emptied your bladder before your examination is also a great help, especially when your doctor is squeezing around in your pelvis, checking the size and consistency of your uterus.

Figure 9 **Taking a cervical smear**

If your uterus is enlarged, or if your ovaries are enlarged or difficult to feel because you are overweight or tense, discuss with your doctor the possibility of having an ultrasound scan of your pelvis. This can reveal uterine fibroids (fibrous growths) or tumours and cysts on the ovaries. Cancer of the ovaries becomes more common during the postmenopausal years and carries a very high risk of death, because if produces few symptoms in the early stages. Ovarian cancer is the fifth deadliest cancer in women and kills twice as many women as cancer of the cervix. It is usually discovered in women over the age of forty-five, at a stage when it has spread extensively. In general, it is a slow-growing cancer that is not diagnosed until late. An ultrasound scan can help to discover growths on the ovaries in the earlier and more curable stages. The more frequent use of ultrasound scans of the pelvis to check the ovaries in women over forty-five should reduce the currently pessimistic statistics for ovarian cancer. Table 1 gives an overview of tests your doctor will probably perform or arrange and what he or she will be looking for.

Figure 10 **The female reproductive tract (front view)**

Figure 11 **The female reproductive tract (side view)**

SPECIAL TESTS

Ideally, all women should begin to have biennial mammograms, or breast X-rays, at the age of forty years. The reason for this is that mammograms can detect breast cancer before a palpable lump has developed, and increase the rate of early detection. Early detection of breast cancer increases survival rates.

At the very least, you should have a mammogram at the time of menopause, if you are over forty, and especially before beginning HRT. This is because if you have a tiny, undiagnosed cancer lurking in your breast, HRT could stimulate its growth. Thus, it is important to rule out the presence of a breast cancer before beginning HRT, and a mammogram is the most accurate means of doing this. Your doctor will examine your breasts very carefully for signs of cancer, but even the best doctor in the world can miss a tiny cancer because it is just too small to feel. A good-quality low-radiation-dose mammogram can reveal very tiny cancers, as small as one to two millimetres in size, long before you or your doctor would be able to feel it. In Sweden, studies have proven that routine screening of women aged forty-five years and over with regular mammograms can reduce deaths from breast cancer by up to 60 per cent.

In addition to mammograms, a menopausal woman should have a bone mineral density (BMD) test to measure the strength of her bones. This will enable your doctor to assess whether you are showing signs of osteoporosis and, if you are, to recommend treatment to try to rebuild bone, or at least to slow bone loss. Ideally, you should have a BMD test done when you reach menopause and at regular intervals thereafter (see page 39).

Other tests that should be performed include a complete blood count to check for anaemia, as well as blood tests to check your liver function and measure your levels of follicle-stimulating hormone (FSH), oestrogen, blood sugar, and cholesterol. If you have a past history of thrombosis (the formation of clots in the blood vessels), then blood should be taken for a clotting factor profile.

TABLE 1

A MENOPAUSE EXAMINATION CHECKLIST

This table provides you with a general checklist of important tests that are often performed at menopause, together with what the doctor is looking for when doing them. Your doctor will decide if any special tests, such as blood tests or pelvic ultrasound, are needed in your individual case.

EXAMINATON	WHAT THE DOCTOR LOOKS FOR
The Physical Examination	
Heart, blood pressure, blood vessels	High or low blood pressure; signs of cardiovascular disease; varicose veins.
Weight	Underweight; obesity.
Thyroid gland	Enlargement; lumps. Under- or over-activity can be confirmed with a blood test for thyroid function.
Breasts	Lumps; thickening; skin or nipple changes.
Abdomen	Swelling; tenderness.
Pelvic examination	Size of pelvic organs; condition of ovaries; signs of cancer, prolapse of uterus or bladder, vaginal atrophy.
Special Tests	
Cervical smear	Cancerous or pre-cancerous cells in the cervix.
Mammogram	Very early signs of breast cancer.
Bone mineral density test (BMD)	Signs of osteoporosis.
Blood count; blood tests for oestrogen, follicle-stimulating hormone (FSH), blood sugar, liver function, cholesterol level	Blood oestrogen level; signs of metabolic disorders.
Urinalysis	Signs of infection, kidney disease.
Pelvic ultrasound	Signs of disease of the uterus and/or ovaries. Pelvic ultrasound is useful for women in whom pelvic examination is difficult, uncomfortable, or inconclusive.

FOLLOW-UP VISITS

All postmenopausal women should see their doctors annually. If you are using only natural therapies, such as herbs and nutritional supplements, then the frequency of follow-up visits will vary, depending on your symptoms. However, an annual check-up should still be done. Using natural therapies is more of a self-help enterprise than HRT is. Unless you are working with a nutritionally oriented physician, you may prefer to visit your local health food store or a naturopathic physician for advice about adjusting your dosage of vitamins, for example. You will also find Chapters 6 and 7, which discuss natural therapies and nutrition in detail, to be invaluable. The material in these chapters is based on my many years of clinical research into the use of herbs, vitamins, minerals, and essential fatty acids to relieve menopausal symptoms.

If you decide to try hormone replacement therapy, you will probably make this decision during your second visit to the doctor, at which time you and your doctor can review and discuss the results of all your tests. You may decide to start taking HRT immediately, or you may feel you need time to think about it, to seek a second opinion, or to sort out your feelings about HRT. The most pressing reason to begin oestrogen replacement wthout delay would be a poor result on your bone mineral density (BMD) test, which would mean that you are at high risk of developing osteoporosis.

If you decide to take HRT, monitor its effects by keeping a weekly record of the symptoms on your oestrogen deficiency chart (see page 21). After you start HRT, your doctor will probably recommend follow-up appointments after two months, six months, and twelve months, and thereafter at twelve-month intervals. This will enable your doctor to fine-tune your HRT to suit your individual needs. A general physical examination, cervical smear, and mammogram should be repeated every twelve months. If the results of your initial BMD test are satisfactory, this test can be repeated every three to five years. If the test shows a low mineral content in your bones, you should have additional BMD tests done every one to two years.

If irregular, unexplained vaginal bleeding occurs twelve months after menopause, whether you are on HRT or not, a curettage of the uterus or a hysteroscopy should be done by a gynaecologist. Some experts feel that all women on long-term HRT should have more than a cervical smear every twelve months. They recommend the addition of a test called an endometrial biopsy, in which a sample of cells from the lining of the uterus is taken and examined under a microscope. This is done to check for pre-cancerous cells in the uterus, above the cervix. It can easily be done at the time of your regular cervical smear.

I hope that after reading about all the various aspects of your anatomy and biochemistry that require regular surveillance you will be more inspired and less forgetful about making your visits to the doctor. I am horrified when I see a woman on HRT who has never had a breast examination or a mammogram, or a woman who believes, because she is using only natural therapies for menopause, that she no longer needs an a regular cervical smear. I have also met older women who feel that their doctors are not interested in checking their breasts and genital organs, and who feel embarrassed to ask about it. This is sad – and also potentially dangerous. To safeguard your health in your menopausal and postmenopausal years, it is more important than ever before that you find a sympathetic doctor whom you can trust and with whom you can communicate.

CHAPTER FOUR

EVERYTHING YOU WILL EVER NEED TO KNOW ABOUT HORMONE REPLACEMENT THERAPY

Hormone replacement therapy is an option for every menopausal woman, but the decision to take it should be her own, based on accurate information and her individual lifestyle and health requirements. In addition, different HRT regimens are appropriate for different women. Some women need to take oestrogen only; others require combination HRT, including both oestrogen and progesterone. Hormones are often taken in tablet form, but some women fare better using other methods of administration, such as patches or injections.

In order to make an informed decision about taking HRT, you need to know about all the choices available to you, and their comparative advantages and disadvantages. In this chapter I will provide you with complete information about all the options available today, so that you will be able to make the decision that is right for you.

OESTROGEN

The basic element of any programme of hormone replacement therapy is oestrogen. This powerful sex hormone exerts effects throughout the body. Among other things, it helps to keep your skin soft, your bones strong, and your arteries clear.

Oestrogen is available in different forms. One of the first and most important issues to understand, if you are considering hormone replacement therapy, is the distinction between natural and synthetic oestrogen. There is a tremendous difference between the two.

SYNTHETIC OESTROGEN

Synthetic oestrogens are manufactured in laboratories. They are chemically foreign to the body's metabolic systems and so are not easily broken down by the body's natural enzymes. Consequently, they can accumulate in the body, causing them to exert stronger effects than the natural oestrogens. Synthetic oestrogens can also cause metabolic changes in the liver, leading to an increased incidence of side-effects such as fluid retention, blood clots, aching legs, and high blood pressure. I prefer to avoid giving synthetic oestrogens to menopausal and postmenopausal women. Natural oestrogens are so much safer and are now widely available. In addition to ethinyl oestradiol, which is marketed under various brand names, synthetic oestrogens include quinestrol and diethylstilbestrol (better known as DES).

NATURAL OESTROGEN

Natural oestrogen is mostly developed in laboratories, where an exact chemical replica of your ovaries' oestrogen is cleverly synthesized. Although it may seem like a paradox to say that something natural can be synthesized, the important thing is that the end product is a hormone identical to the one produced by your own ovaries. Your body treats the synthesized natural oestrogen exactly as it would your ovarian oestrogen – it cannot tell any difference.

One popular type of natural oestrogen, called Premarin, is extracted from the urine of pregnant mares. Premarin contains a mixture of natural humanlike oestrogen (oestrone sulphate) and some more potent equine (horse) oestrogens. (So I suppose you could say that, strictly speaking, Premarin is natural only for horses!) In general, Premarin is an excellent form of replacement oestrogen for menopausal women. However, because of its potency it can cause metabolic changes in the liver. For this reason, it should probably not be used by women who are obese, who smoke cigarettes, or who suffer from high blood pressure, high cholesterol, or varicose veins.

The most common truly natural oestrogens are piperazine oestrone sulphate (sold under the brand name Harmogen) and oestradiol (Progynova, Climaval, Estraderm, Evaril and others). These natural oestrogens are familiar to our bodies' metabolic systems and are easily broken down into forms that can be readily excreted by the liver and kidneys once they have been utilized and have done their job. They do not accumulate in the body and are therefore less likely to cause side-effects than the synthetic oestrogens are. For these reasons, all women on HRT should be using the safer, natural oestrogens.

Because natural oestrogens are readily metabolized (broken down) by the body, if you take them in tablet form you may need to take them twice daily (at twelve-hour intervals) to maintain adequate blood levels of oestrogen at all times. It is not uncommon to see women on a once-a-day regimen of natural oestrogen tablets who complain of hot flushes, vaginal dryness, fatigue, and other symptoms of oestrogen deficiency. Blood tests often reveal that such women have inadequate levels of oestrogen. In such cases, women usually experience great improvement if they take their oestrogen tablets at twelve-hour rather than twenty-four-hour intervals.

OESTROGENS MOST OFTEN USED FOR HRT

Table 2 lists some of the oestrogen tablets most commonly prescribed for HRT. As you can see, the daily dosages of oestrogen tablets vary considerably in amount, depending on how rapidly your enzymes break them down, as well as on which brand of oestrogen is prescribed. For example, Harmogen (oestrone) is three times stronger than Ovestin (oestriol), and Progynova (oestradiol) is ten times stronger than Ovestin (oestriol). In all cases, you must be guided by your own doctor in finding your required dose. Perimenopausal women (women in the years leading up to, during, and just after the final menstruation, roughly aged forty-five to fifty-five) still produce their own hormones erratically and generally need higher doses of HRT than women in their later fifties or sixties.

TABLE 2

OESTROGEN TABLETS AND DOSES

Brand Name	Chemical Name	Type	Daily Dose Range (mg)	Daily Minimum Dose to Prevent Osteoporosis (mg)
Premarin	Conjugated equine oestrogen	Semi-natural	0.3–1.25	0.625
Progynova Climaval	Oestradiol valerate	Natural	1–4	2.0
Harmogen	Piperazine oestrone sulphate	Natural	0.625–2.5	1.25
Ovestin	Oestriol	Natural	1–4	2.0
Kliofem	Oestradiol	Natural	1–4	2.0

SOME NEW INFORMATION ON OESTROGEN

The female hormone oestrogen is naturally produced in the body in at least three forms. The first two forms, oestrone (E1) and oestradiol (E2) are relatively potent oestrogens that can relieve menopausal symptoms very well, but can also produce side-effects and may possibly increase breast cancer risk if they are given in high doses or for a prolonged period of time (say more than five years). E2 is made by the ovary. E1 is made from E2 and also from the hormone called androstenedione which is a male hormone made in the ovary and the adrenal gland.

The third form of naturally produced body oestrogen is oestriol (E3) and this is produced from the other oestrogens, E E2. Because oestriol (E3) is less potent than the first two form oestrogen some researchers believe it is less likely to stimulate the breast and uterine lining (endometrium) in an unfavourable way. Oestriol is available in Britain under the brand name of Ovestin, in the form of both tablets and a vaginal cream. For women who are worried about using the stronger oestrogens (oestradiol and oestrone), the weaker oestriol form of oestrogen may be safer and produce less side-effects.

Alvin H. Follinstad, MD, of Albuquerque, New Mexico, states that oestriol does not lose its identity when given by mouth as does oestradiol.[1] It remains oestriol. A dose of 4 mg of oestriol is the equivalent of 0.6 mg of Premarin and is just as effective. Dr Follinstad states that if prescribing oestrogen to high-risk patients, oestriol will pose the least risk.

I personally do not prescribe the Premarin brand of oestrogen, which contains a mixture of oestrone and equine (horse) oestrogens, as the pregnant mares and foals involved in producing Premarin are subjected to suffering and cruelty. Other natural forms of oestrogen are easily available which do not involve any cruelty to animals.

TRI-OESTROGEN

Tri-oestrogen is used by some doctors in America and is formulated to contain all the three naturally occurring oestrogens in a safe and effective way. Tri-oestrogen replacement therapy was developed by Dr Jonathan Wright, MD, of Kent, Washington, after he conducted tests to measure the blood levels and urinary excretion of the three natural forms of oestrogen in his patients. He then developed a compound with the proportion of 80 per cent oestriol, ten per cent oestrone and 10 per cent oestradiol. He found that a dose of 2.5 to 5 mg of tri-oestrogen effectively relieves menopausal symptoms such as hot flushes, sweating and vaginal dryness.

A type of tri-oestrogen is available in Britain under the brand name Hormonin. However, it contains different proportions of the three oestrogens compared to the compound developed by Dr Wright. Hormonin is made up of approximately 12 per cent oestriol, 62 per cent oestrone and 26 per cent oestradiol, and may be preferable for women with more severe symptoms of oestrogen deficiency.

Dr Stephen Corson, MD, from the Philadephia Fertility Institute, has had a decade of experience with oestrogen patches (transdermal oestrogen). His clinical findings are that oestrogen patches are as effective as oral oestrogen in controlling many of the untoward metabolic changes associated with menopause, such as elevated cholesterol and lowered calcium levels. Oestrogen patches are safer for women with liver problems, high blood pressure, varicose veins or a past history of blood clots.

While I was in Kansas City, Missouri, I met a very interesting female pharmacist by the name of Lisa Everett. Lisa is a compounding pharmacist, which means that she can mix tailor-made combinations of natural hormones for individual patients according to the doctor's prescription. She has been doing this for many years and can tailor varying doses of oestrogen/progesterone combinations in the form of suppositories, capsules, creams and troches. Troches are square-shaped tablets containing one or more hormones and flavouring. They are slowly dissolved in the oral cavity between the gum and cheek and are sometimes called lozenges or pastilles. Troches can deliver hormones across the mucosal lining of the cheek and into the bloodstream, whereas, with swallowing, the hormones may be destroyed or more poorly absorbed.

Using troche technology it is possible to customize women's HRT by varying the types and amount of hormones. For example, women with a higher risk of breast cancer can be given only oestriol (E3) along with natural progesterone to relieve menopausal symptoms. Oestriol has not been linked with cancer increases in recent studies and is a far safer choice for some high-risk women; if preferred, a low-dose oestrogen patch (say 25 to 50 strength) is also safer.

For women with a higher risk of cardiovascular disease the troche can contain more oestradiol and oestrone for increased protection. Troches can be customized to contain all of the three naturally occurring oestrogens in varying proportions according to the doctor's prescription.

In America, natural progesterone is sometimes prescribed in the form of troches or vaginal pessaries to help alleviate conditions such as premenstrual syndrome, postnatal depression and heavy painful periods. Natural progesterone can also be of help for endometriosis. Progesterone is a hormone produced by the ovaries in the second half of the menstrual cycle, after ovulation has occurred and is necessary for pregnancy to occur. It was first isolated in 1934 by a number of researchers as a white crystalline powder which is odourless, stable in air and not very water soluble. Today natural progesterone is made from extracts of yams or soyabeans and is chemically identical to the hormone produced naturally by the ovaries. The term 'natural progesterone' is often confused with synthetic progestogens. Synthetic progestogens are derivatives of progesterone used in medications like the oral contraceptive pill, under various brand names. Although the difference in the chemical structure of natural progesterone and synthetic progestogens is slight, their effects in the body are very different and these medications cannot be used interchangeably. Synthetic progestogens can inhibit ovulation, thus suppressing the body's output of its own natural progesterone. This is not important in menopausal women who no longer ovulate anyway; however, in younger women with premenstrual syndrome this is not helpful, as what they need is more natural progesterone. The synthetic progestogens fit on to the cell receptors for progesterone and this means that any natural progesterone, either produced by the body or prescribed by a doctor, cannot fit on to these receptors; thus synthetic progestogens block the effects of natural progesterone. This is why synthetic progestogens are not effective treatments for premenstrual syndrome. When synthetic progestogens were developed more than thirty-five year ago, the difference between the natural progesterone and the synthetic progestogens was not clearly understood. Some confusion still often exists in the medical profession today, although the difference between the natural and synthetic progesterones is now well documented. In particular the synthetic progestogens are effective for endometriosis, heavy painful periods and contraception, but will not help women with premenstrual syndrome; indeed synthetic progestogens usually make premenstrual syndrome worse. It is interesting to note that natural progesterone is converted into other natural steroid hormones in the adrenal gland (synthetic progestogens are not), and these steroid hormones produce beneficial effects upon mood disorders and fatigue. Furthermore, all naturally produced steroid hormones, including cortisone, oestrogen, progesterone and androgens, are made in the ovaries and adrenal glands from cholesterol. Thus, women who eliminate all fats from the diet, especially if very underweight, will not produce sufficient sex hormones and may suffer with a diverse range of hormonal disorders. So some eggs and fresh seafood and low-fat dairy foods (unless allergic) should be eaten regularly to keep your hormones and libido healthy!

For premenstrual syndrome, natural progesterone in the form of troches or vaginal pessaries in a dose of 400 mg (approximately) is given during the two weeks before the onset of menstrual bleeding.

In the United Kingdom, Dr Katharina Dalton pioneered the use of natural progesterones for premenstrual syndrome, postnatal depresson and other hormonal imbalances. For further information on the availability and use of natural progesterone you could try contacting her office at 60 Wimpole St., London W1. Alternatively you or your doctor can obtain information on natural progesterone and oestrogen troches from two American compounding pharmacies: Lisa Everett, pharmacist, O'Brien Pharmacy, 4320 Wornall Road, Kansas City, Missouri, 64111, USA. Phone 001-816-5316763. Apthorp Pharmacy, 2201 Broadway at 78th Street, New York, New York, 10024. Phone 001-212-8773480. A doctor can order drugs from abroad wth a prescription.

PROGESTERONE – THE BALANCING HORMONE

In addition to oestrogen, the ovary also makes the female sex hormone progesterone. Progesterone balances the effects of oestrogen on the uterus and is necessary to produce regular periods.

If a woman with a uterus is taking replacement oestrogen, it is now universally accepted that she must also take progesterone for at least ten to twelve days every calendar month in order to prevent uterine cancer. If oestrogen is taken alone, there is an increased risk of cancer of the uterus. It is most reassuring to know that if a woman on HRT takes progesterone in addition to oestrogen, her risk of uterine cancer actually *decreases*, to the point where it is lower than that of a woman who is not on HRT!

Expert opinion is somewhat divided as to the necessity of adding some progesterone to oestrogen replacement for a woman without a uterus (a woman who has undergone a hysterectomy). Some studies show that progesterone taken for twelve days every calendar month may exert a protective role against breast cancer, but this has not been categorically proven and debate on the subject continues.

Currently, the progesterone tablets that are commonly used along with oestrogen in HRT contain synthetic progesterone. Synthetic forms of progesterone are called progestogens. Progestogens are not as good as natural progesterone, because they do not quite fit the progesterone receptors on your cells. However, they do still balance the effect of oestrogen on the uterus.

Some of the progestogens currently used can have adverse

TABLE 3 PROGESTERONES

Note: **Progestagen** = Synthetic progesterone, **Progesterone** = Natural progesterone

Brand Name	Chemical Name	Type	Daily Dosage (mg)	Advantages	Disadvantages
Provera tablets	Medroxy-progesterone acetate	Synthetic	2.5–10	Does not cause adverse effects on cholesterol.	May cause PMS-type symptoms in excessive dosage.
Primolut N Micronor Noriday tablets	Norethisterone	Synthetic	0.35–5	May reduce breast tenderness.	May exert masculine effects, but generally less than Levonorgestrel. May cause adverse effect on cholesterol.
Microval Norgeston tablets	Levonorgestrel	Synthetic	0.03–0.09		May cause adverse effect on cholesterol. May exert masculine effects.
Micronised progesterone tablets	Not available in Britain	Natural	200–300	No recognised side-effects. No ill-effects on cholesterol.	Expensive. Absorption may be poor.
Duphaston tablets	Dydrogestrone	Semi-natural (neutral)	10–20	Generally fewer side-effects. Does not cause adverse effects on cholesterol.	May cause bloating and fluid retention in susceptible women.
Progesterone patches	Norethisterone (synthetic). Natural form not available in most countries.	Natural or synthetic	Not determined	Fewer side-effects. Most natural way of giving progesterone.	Skin sensitivity. Breakthrough bleeding.
Androcur tablets	Cyproterone acetate	Synthetic	12.5–100	Reduces facial hair and acne. improves skin texture.	If dose too high may cause fatigue, depression and loss of libido.
Proluton Depot injection	Hydroxy progesterone hexanoate	Semi-natural (neutral)	Not applicable. Give one injection every 4–6 weeks in buttocks.	Generally no side-effects.	Injection site may be tender for several days.
Progesterone troches	May be difficult to obtain in Britain.	Natural	200–600	No recognised side-effects. No ill-effects on cholesterol.	Expensive. Use under doctor's supervision.
Cyclogest suppositories	Progesterone	Natural	200–400, 1 – 2 times daily rectally or vaginally	Less side-effects. No ill-effects on cholesterol.	May cause rectal or vaginal irritation.

effects on cholesterol levels, which may reduce the beneficial effect of oestrogen on the blood vessels (see Table 3). While the debate continues, it is best to be guided by your doctor and use a progestogen such as Duphaston (dydrogesterone) or Provera (medroxyprogesterone acetate) that will not have an ill effect on your cholesterol balance. These progestogens can also be found in the tablets Femoston (oestradiol and dydrogesterone), Improvera (oestrone and medroxyprogesterone acetate) and Tridestra (oestradiol and medroxyprogesterone acetate).

Some women refuse to take any progestogen tablets because they can cause such annoying side-effects as irritability, depression, headaches, weight gain, bloating, and pelvic pain. If the side-effects are intolerable, progestogen tablets can safely be omitted for a woman who has had a hysterectomy. If you have a uterus, you can discuss with your doctor the option of omitting progestogens. Another option for a woman who still has her uterus is to take semi-natural progesterone injections (available under the brand name of Proluton Depot) given as one injection every 28 days. In my experience, progesterone injections are very well tolerated and free of side-effects, although because they are oily, some tenderness may be felt in the buttocks, the site of the injection. Progesterone injections act in a similar way to progestogen tablets in regulating the menstrual cycle and bringing on regular monthly bleeding. Natural progesterone has very few side-effects and is better tolerated than the synthetic progestogens, which may cause side-effects in susceptible women. In particular, natural progesterone does not cause the depression or unpleasant moods that progestogens sometimes do.

Natural progesterone is made from soyabeans and yams. The required dosages are quite high, ranging from 200 to 400 milligrams daily for ten to twelve days out of every calendar month. These higher doses are necessary because natural progesterone is not as potent as the synthetic progestogens are. The main drawbacks of natural progesterone tablets, suppositories, and injections are that they are relatively expensive and some doctors are unfamiliar with their use. However, if you feel great while taking oestrogen alone, only to find that once you add in the synthetic progestogen your mental and physical well-being deteriorate, then natural progesterone may hold the key to health and happiness for you. If your doctor is unfamiliar with natural progesterone products, you can encourage him or her to contact the Madison Pharmacy Association in Madison, Wisconsin, or O'Brien Pharmacy in Kansas City, Missouri, for more information. These companies sell pure natural micronized progesterone in a variety of forms, including tablets, capsules, suppositories, creams, and troches (small lozenges designed to dissolve when held against the inside of the cheek). *Micronized* progesterone is progesterone that has been broken into tiny particles so that it is better absorbed and utilized.

If you find you are unable to tolerate the side-effects that progestogens or even natural progesterone may produce, you can ask your doctor's permission to leave them out completely, but if you do you should have your endometrium (the lining of your uterus) checked every twelve months with a biopsy or hysteroscopy. As a last resort, if you feel very unwell without oestrogen replacement, and yet feel even worse on progestogens, a hysterectomy could be a possibility. This is a drastic measure, but it is a possible option if you are very worried about increasing your risk of uterine cancer from unopposed oestrogen replacement.

TAKING ORAL HRT

The most widely used and best-known form of HRT is the oral, or tablet, form, and most research has been done using this form. Most women who take HRT are happy to take tablets of oestrogen and progesterone on a cyclical basis, in much the same fashion that oral contraceptive pills are taken. Hormone tablets can be taken according to many different time and dosage schedules. Your doctor will work with you to determine the appropriate timing and dosage for you, depending on your response to HRT and, to a certain extent, on your lifestyle.

One of the most important points to understand about HRT is that if you still have a uterus – that is, if you have not had a hysterectomy – you must also take progesterone in addition to oestrogen for at least ten to twelve days out of every calendar month. This will ensure regular monthly bleeding and greatly reduce your risk of developing cancer of the uterus. In fact, there is less of a risk of this type of cancer in women on combination HRT than there is in women who take no hormone replacement at all. Oestrogen tablets are often taken once or twice daily for twenty-one or twenty-five days, with a five-day break between courses, and with progesterone tablets being taken for the last twelve days of the course (see Tables 1 and 2). Menstrual bleeding usually occurs during the five-day break from the oestrogen tablets. Alternatively, the oestrogen tablets can be taken continually every day, with progesterone being taken for the first twelve days of every calendar month (see Figure 12).

CAN MENSTRUAL BLEEDING BE AVOIDED?

My catch phrase for the 1990s is 'designer HRT'. This refers to the fact that today every woman who wants HRT can have it tailor-made to suit her unique needs. A lot of older postmenopausal women stop HRT because they don't want monthly menstrual bleeding. This is a pity, as 'designer HRT' can reduce or completely eliminate menstrual bleeding.

Some women feel better having a five-day break from oestrogen, but if you don't, there is no harm in taking oestrogen every day. In fact, taking oestrogen every day is better for your bones and blood vessels. There is no risk, provided you also take your progesterone tablets for at least twelve days of each calendar month (see Figure 12).

Nowadays, older women are often prescribed both oestrogen

Figure 12 **Hormone tablet schedules**

and progesterone tablets to be taken every day without a break, which completely eliminates menstrual bleeding. If any spotting or breakthrough bleeding occurs on this programme, you may take a seven-day break from the oestrogen and progesterone tablets every three months, which enables your uterus to shed any build-up lining in the form of a light menstrual period. Some women feel more comfortable having menstrual bleeding every three months or so, seeing it as a kind of 'spring cleaning' for the uterus, after which they often feel better.

If you are a postmenopausal woman over the age of sixty-five and it is thought necessary for you to begin taking HRT for the first time to slow the progression of osteoporosis, you may take a small dose of oestrogen continuously with no breaks at all. In such cases, light menstrual bleeding can be brought on only two or three times a year by the addition of a two-week course of progesterone tablets. This reduces the annoyance of regular monthly bleeding. Single HRT pills that combine the two hormones oestrogen and progestogen are available under the brand names Kliofem (oestradiol plus norethisterone) and Premique (conjugated oestrogens and medroxyprogesterone) and are taken every day without a break, eliminating menstrual bleeding completely.

A small-dose oestrogen patch is a very safe and gentle way of giving HRT to older women.

EVERY WOMAN IS DIFFERENT

One woman's oestrogen replacement needs may be two to four times higher than another's. Curiously enough, it is often the woman with a thin, lean build who needs greater amounts of oestrogen. This is because such women tend to have very little production of oestrogen from their fatty tissues. Furthermore, it is the thin, fine-boned woman who has a greater risk of osteoporosis and may need to take a greater amount of oestrogen to prevent this.

Modern-day HRT has become so safe and effective in the prevention of many problems that every menopausal woman should be aware of its benefits. As long as no medical risks exist, HRT is an option about which you are entitled to make your own informed decision. However, it is true that menopausal women differ in their need for HRT. Some women say that they cannot live without it – they feel ancient, decrepit, and lifeless without oestrogen in their bodies – while others hardly seem to notice when their ovaries finally stop producing oestrogen. There are also some menopausal and postmenopausal women who actually feel worse on HRT, no matter what different forms and dosages are tried. Such was the story of Mandy, a big-boned, somewhat obese fifty-five-year-old woman who complained that she had gained over fifteen pounds and experienced fluid retention, aching legs, and fatigue since beginning HRT three years before. Her blood pressure was elevated and her legs were bulging with varicose veins. Mandy had started taking hormone tablets at the time of her natural menopause, without any blood tests or a bone mineral density (BMD) check being done to assess her individual need for oestrogen. I checked her bone mineral density and found it to be excellent. She had no risk factors for osteoporosis or heart disease. In fact, her mother had lived to the age of ninety-eight with no trace of either osteoporosis or cardiovascular disease.

Thus, Mandy did not need to take HRT. Indeed, in her case, its side-effects were greater than its benefits. She stopped HRT and six months later had lost thirteen pounds, regained her normal blood pressure, and generally felt much better. All Mandy needed was a doctor's permission to stop HRT, with the assurance that her bones and blood vessels would be checked regularly to make sure that she was not showing signs of developing osteoporosis or cardiovascular disease. In my opinion, Mandy was someone who did better without HRT. Menopausal women should not be made to feel that they must take HRT or else terrible things will happen to them. Rather, they should be given the information they need to make an informed decision. The merits of HRT vary for different individuals.

HORMONE REPLACEMENT THERAPY AFTER HYSTERECTOMY

Approximately one in five women in the United Kingdom have a hysterectomy by the age of fifty. HRT is simpler for women who have had a hysterectomy. In such cases, experts agree that progestogen tablets are not necessary. An exception here is the woman who had a past history of endometriosis, a disorder in which cells from the endometrium (the lining of the uterus) are found growing outside the uterus, in the abdominal cavity. Endometriosis can be reactivated by oestrogen replacement unless sufficient progesterone is taken to balance the oestrogen therapy. Women with a past history of endometriosis (whether they have had a hysterectomy or not) should take low-dose progesterone tablets continually along with oestrogen. If a woman has no past history of endometriosis, she can take oestrogen by itself in the form of oestrogen tablets, patches, injections or implants.

If the ovaries are conserved during hysterectomy in a premenopausal woman, they will usually function normally for many years after the operation. However, menopause may still arrive two to three years earlier than it would have otherwise. It is not uncommon for a woman to find that after hysterectomy, her ovaries do not work as well as they did before. She may complain of symptoms of oestrogen deficiency. This is because the removal of the uterus can cause a reduction in the blood supply to the ovaries, and thus the ovaries no longer pump out adequate amounts of sex hormones. If this happens, a woman can accurately be called premenopausal.

If you think this may be the case for you, compute your oestrogen level score (see page 21), and if your score is around 20, ask your doctor for a blood test to measure levels of follicle-stimulating hormone (FSH), oestrogen, and testosterone. If your FSH levels are elevated and your oestrogen and testosterone levels are low, then your body is low in sex hormones. This may produce fatigue, depression, aches and pains, and loss of libido. A significant number of women in this situation find that hormone tablets do not alleviate these symptoms, and that they need to take either oestrogen or oestrogen and testosterone in non-tablet form, such as patches, injections or implants. These may be better absorbed by the body than tablets are. If you try one of these types of HRT, you may find that your mental, physical, and sexual well-being soar to new heights, perhaps even better than before your hysterectomy.

If the ovaries are removed during hysterectomy, the arrival of menopause is abrupt and severe symptoms of oestrogen deficiency often occur. This is particularly noticeable in younger premenopausal women. Thankfully, oestrogen replacement in the form of tablets, patches, injections or implants can stop unpleasant menopausal symptoms. If both ovaries are removed, a woman's testosterone level also may become very low (the ovaries produce testosterone as well as oestrogen), so she may require testosterone replacement in the form of tablets, injections or implants.

If you have had an endometrial ablation, you may still have some remnants of the uterine lining left behind and will need progesterone tablets to balance the effects of your oestrogen replacement therapy on the endometrium. Endometrial ablation is a procedure in which high-frequency radio waves are used to ablate (destroy) the lining of the uterus, with the aim of reducing or stopping menstrual bleeding. (For a discussion of endometrial ablation, see Chapter 5.)

NON-ORAL FORMS OF HRT

Although hormone tablets are the most commonly used type of HRT, they do not suit all menopausal women, either because of the side-effects or because of an inadequate response. It is important for you to be aware of other forms of hormone replacement that are not taken orally, such as injections (unavailable in Britain), patches, and vaginal creams and suppositories. In many countries, including Great Britain, hormones are also available as implants that are inserted into the fat of the buttocks or abdomen. These non-oral forms of hormone replacement are absorbed directly into the bloodstream, bypassing the digestive tract and the liver. This enables the hormones to travel directly to their target cells all over the body, where they exert their effects. After this they travel to the liver, where they are broken down and excreted.

Oral or tablet forms of hormones, on the other hand, must be absorbed from the intestines, and from there travel directly to the liver, where a significant amount of hormone is metabolised (broken down) before it passes into the circulation to travel to its target cells. The effect of hormones is thus weakened by the 'first liver pass'. Furthermore, large amounts of oral hormones passing through the liver tend to induce metabolic changes there, which may produce more side-effects, such as fluid retention and elevated clotting factors in the blood.

If you are on hormone tablets and don't feel well, or find that your symptoms are not relieved, I suggest you ask your doctor about non-oral forms of hormones.

HORMONE INJECTIONS

Hormone injections were first manufactured and used in the 1930s and 1940s by German scientists and doctors. The injectable forms of hormones have proven to be popular among European women since the 1950s. Unfortunately, natural oestrogen in an injectable form is not available in Britain. In the United States and Australia hormone injections have been used only to a small degree, probably because they are not promoted at all by drug companies and clinical research material on their use is not widely accessible. Furthermore, some doctors feel that absorption from these injections is erratic, producing large fluctuations in the levels of hormones in the blood. Nevertheless, hormone injections continue to be popular in Europe.

I feel that there is a role for injectable forms of natural hormones. Although I do not think they should be the first choice for all women, I have found that for some they can be more suitable than tablet forms. I myself am a migraine sufferer and cannot take tablet forms of oestrogen. Indeed, oestrogen tablets – both synthetic and natural forms – greatly aggravated my migraines, producing classic visual auras including flashing lights and blurred vision. After a hysterectomy for fibroids, I found that my ovaries became premenopausal and did not produce sufficient amounts of oestrogen. I began receiving injections of natural oestrogen into my buttocks every two weeks and found that for me they really did the trick. They relieved my fatigue, loss of enthusiasm, aches and pains, and frequent headaches. My shrinking breasts became fuller, my libido returned, and my acne disappeared. I found that the injections produced a steady release of that wonderful hormone oestrogen into my blood, provided I received them on a regular fortnightly basis. To my relief, they were not painful. (Doctors are generally the biggest cowards and worst patients of all!) I did find that proper injection technique is most important; the needle should be placed deeply into the upper outer part of the buttock, which is the area with the greatest amount of fat. With this technique, the injection produces a slight dull stinging sensation lasting five to ten minutes, which is a small price to pay for the wonderful mental and physical well-being that the oestrogen provides. Injectable forms of the natural hormones oestrogen, progesterone and testosterone are summarized in Table 4.

I first learned of oestrogen injections when a remarkable New York journalist popped into my surgery one day to get her 'fix', as she called it, of injectable oestrogen (in Australia this is called Primogyn Depot). Melanie was a woman in her early sixties, but she looked at least twenty years younger. She related in her vivacious, extroverted way that she had been having one injection every month since her hysterectomy thirty years before. She was in excellent health, and her bone mineral density test did not reveal any signs of osteoporosis. This episode increased my interest in the usefulness of hormone injections, and I am eternally grateful for this to Melanie; hormone injections were not discussed at all in the curriculum at the medical school or at the teaching hospitals where I received my training.

HOW HORMONE INJECTIONS TRANSFORMED TWO WOMEN'S LIVES

Any doctor concerned with the well-being of menopausal women will realize that every woman is an individual and that it may be necessary to try different forms and dosages of HRT before physical and mental well-being can be restored. Miranda, age fifty-one, came to see me in a very distressed state. She had been on a standard dose of hormone tablets for two years but still complained of vaginal dryness and itching, poor libido, headaches, mood changes, insomnia, loss of confidence, and black depression. She was very frightened by these uncharacteristic changes in herself and felt she was becoming dependent on sedatives. Her psychiatrist – a man – told her that it could not be her hormones playing up, as she was on oestrogen tablets. He told her she should give up working and concentrate more on her husband's needs. He also prescribed a large dose of anti-depressant drugs and told her that she would need them to lead a normal life.

TABLE 4 **INJECTABLE NATURAL HORMONES**

Type of hormone	Frequency of injection	Uses
Oestrogen (oestradiol valerate)	One injection every two weeks.	1 Menopause and premenopause; premature menopause. 2 Oestrogen deficiency after hysterectomy. 3 Oestrogen deficiency after surgical removal of the ovaries. 4 Some severe cases of premenstrual syndrome (PMS) and postnatal depression.
Progesterone (hydroxy progesterone hexanoate)	One injection every four weeks at mid-cycle.	1 Menopause in women unable to tolerate oral progestagens. 2 Premenstrual syndrome. 3 Postnatal depression.
Oestrogen and testosterone combination	One injection every four to six weeks. Some women only require one injection two to three times per year.	1 Best used on a temporary or intermittent basis to treat difficult menopausal symptoms, hormonal deficiency after hysterectomy or removal of the ovaries. 2 Loss of libido, frigidity and poor marital relationships. 3 Severe postnatal depression. Note: Testosterone is a male hormone and if excessive doses are used, masculine changes may occur, e.g. increased facial hair and deepening of the voice.

Note: Progesterone must always be given with oestrogen in women who still have a uterus.

Miranda had scratched her vagina and vulva to the point that the area had developed fissures (dry cracks), and would often bleed after attempts at sexual intercourse. Her blood tests revealed lowish levels of oestrogen, so I asked her to double her dose of oestrogen tablets and use a vaginal oestrogen cream. After three months on this increased dosage, she returned complaining that her migraines had worsened and that she had experienced only a slight improvement in the vaginal dryness and itching. Her fits of deep depression persisted and her marital situation had deteriorated. I then suggested that her liver was probably very active in breaking down the oestrogen tablets, so that only small amounts of oestrogen were getting past her liver to the rest of her body, which was still crying out for oestrogen. We decided to try a course of natural oestrogen and testosterone injections (see Table 4). This was injected every four weeks, and Miranda took a course of progesterone tablets for ten days out of every month to ensure that regular menstrual bleeding occurred.

One month after the first injection, Miranda returned asking for another. She was delighted with the results of the first injection, which had given her a 90 per cent improvement in all her symptoms. Her vagina had become moist and responsive, her libido was fantastic, her depression had lifted, and her husband was relieved to rediscover the girl he had married. She felt like socializing again and rejoining her exercise classes, and her mental efficiency at work had improved by leaps and bounds. Miranda received a course of three hormone injections, and then we decided to insert an implant of natural oestrogen and testosterone into the fat of her buttocks. She requires an implant every nine to twelve months, and she has never looked back. Her marriage is thriving, she has thrown out her sedatives and anti--depressants, and she continues to enjoy her high-powered job. This is one of many success stories demonstrating that time, patience, and confidence in using the correct type of HRT for each individual woman will usually work.

Miranda was one of the significant percentage of women who do not find relief from oestrogen deficiency symptoms with oestrogen tablets. These women should not be told patronizingly that they have mental or emotional problems or be made to feel inadequate. Rather, they should be offered alternative forms of HRT such as injections, implants or oestrogen patches. If a doctor is not confident in this area, he or she should give an appropriate referral to a women's Health Centre or Menopause Clinic.

Another interesting story is that of forty-three-year-old Selina, who came to see me because of increasing premenstrual syndrome and a total loss of interest in sex. Selina craved more emotional and romantic attention from her fifty-eight-year-old husband, which he was unwilling to give her because he resented her inability to satisfy his sexual appetite. They had been married when Selina was thirty-two, and things had been perfect until she underwent tubal ligation (surgical sterilization) at the age of thirty-five, after the birth of her second child. From that point on, Selina began to experience gradually increasing symptoms of oestrogen and testosterone deficiency, including sudden mood changes, loss of sexual desire, and a reduction in the amount and frequency of her menstrual bleeding. A sample of Selina's blood revealed low oestrogen and very low testosterone levels, consistent with a premenopausal state. To make matters worse, the amount of sex hormone binding globulin (SHBG) her liver was producing was very high. Sex hormone binding globulin is a protein in the blood that binds to and carries the sex hormones oestrogen, progesterone, and testosterone in the bloodstream. Sex hormones are inactive when they are bound to sex hormone binding globulin, so the presence of large amounts of SHBG reduces the active role that sex hormones can play in your body. This was Selina's dilemma: low amounts of sex hormones and a high amount of sex hormone binding globulin circulating around in her body. She didn't stand a chance of feeling sexy, and things could only get worse as she got closer to menopause.

Selina and I designed a six-month programme of oestrogen and progesterone tablets for her, but she returned after four months, saying that her premenstrual irritability and sexual disinterest persisted. We then began a six-month course of monthly natural hormone depot injections. Selina received an injection of oestrogen and testosterone (known as Primodian Depot in Australia) at the end of every menstrual period, and one oestrogen injection (known as Primogyn Depot in Australia) and one progesterone injection (available as Proluton Depot in the UK) on the sixteenth day of every menstrual cycle. This produced a dramatic improvement in her mental, physical, and sexual well-being. Her husband could hardly keep up with this newly energetic and sexual woman. The combination of these three injections, containing natural oestrogen, testosterone, and progesterone, had provided Selina's brain, genital organs, and other sexually responsive body cells with sex hormones that her own premenopausal ovaries could not provide. After six months, Selina found a slight increase in facial hair, so we stopped the injections containing testosterone. She eventually opted for an implant of natural oestrogen without any testosterone, as her libido had returned to normal and she did not want any increase in facial hair.

Selina's case illustrates one of the many flexible programmes of 'designer HRT' that can be tried for women with hormonal imbalances in the premenopausal years. The injectable forms of natural hormones are very useful for what I call a 'hormonal crisis', a severe and/or sudden deficiency or imbalance in hormones such as may occur after a hysterectomy, surgical removal of the ovaries, tubal ligation, sudden onset of menopause, premature menopause, a severe medical illness, severe stress, chemotherapy treatment for cancer, or childbirth. Natural hormone injections can truly work wonders, and can prevent a hormonal crisis from leading you into a deep, dark pit; indeed, they usually take you out of the pit quickly and efficiently. Depending on the cause of your problem, you may need them for only three to six months, until your own hormones recover, or you may continue to need oestrogen and find it more convenient to use an oestrogen patch, an oestrogen implant or the more conventional oestrogen tablet.

OESTROGEN PATCHES

Who would ever have thought that one day we would come up with the idea of applying sticky Band-Aids containing oestrogen to our skin to help us remain well and feminine? The idea is here to stay, and women in America, Britain, and Switzerland have been using the patch for about ten years now.

The natural oestrogen in the patch is absorbed through the skin into the bloodstream. One patch can be worn for three to seven days (depending on the brand) on a convenient part of the buttocks or torso (other than the breasts). The site selected should be one where little wrinkling of the skin occurs during movement of the body, such as the abdomen, buttock, or lower back. There is no need to take a break from using the patches. A woman with a uterus should take progesterone tablets also for ten to twelve days every month. We now also have patches containing both oestrogen and progesterone (norethisterone) which are much better for women suffering emotional side-effects from oral progesterone tablets. Progesterone absorbed transdermally (across the skin) is far less likely to cause these emotional side-effects, although bleeding problems are more common.

Suggested application sites of Estraderm patches:
1 & 2 first week
3 & 4 second week
1 & 2 third week

Estraderm 25
Estraderm 50
Estraderm 100

Estraderm patches

Oestrogen patches contain the natural oestrogen oestradiol, and are sold under the brand names Estraderm, Evorel, Fematrix, Menorest, Femseven and Progyna TS. They come in various strengths depending on the brand, including 25, 37.5, 40, 50, 75, 80 and 100. Occasionally the patches can produce local skin irritation and redness because they contain alcohol. To reduce this irritation, after peeling off the patch's adhesive cover, leave the sticky side of the patch exposed to the air for thirty minutes before applying it to your skin. This simple trick will often make a big difference. It helps to change the site of the patch with each successive application, and you can also use a vitamin E or cortisone cream on irritated skin after removing the patch. In a small number of women, the patch produces severe skin irritation and allergy, which necessitates changing to another form of HRT.

When the oestrogen patch first appeared on the scene, there was some scepticism about its ability to be well absorbed into the bloodstream. However, the patches have undergone extensive testing and have been shown to produce very adequate blood levels of oestradiol – indeed, levels similar to those found in younger women not yet approaching menopause, who still have natural menstrual cycles. A recent study reported in the British medical journal *Lancet* produced very exciting news about the ability of the oestrogen patch to reduce calcium loss from the spinal vertebrae and hipbones. The 50mcg oestrogen patch, which contains 4 milligrams of oestradiol, was found to be just as effective as tablet forms of oestrogen in the prevention of osteoporosis.[2] The oestrogen patch is a very safe way for you to achieve constant and normal levels of oestrogen in your blood. Because the oestrogen is absorbed through the skin and directly into the bloodstream instead of through the digestive tract, it is able to reach your cells before it is broken down by the liver. Thus, smaller doses of oestrogen can be used and side-effects due to metabolic changes in the liver are far less likely. This makes the patch excellent for women with high blood pressure, fluid retention, bloating, varicose veins, obesity, and a past history of clots or thrombosis.

Take the case of Alice, a sixty-two-year-old woman who had been told that she could never take oestrogen because she had suffered two serious blood clots in her leg, one after her hysterectomy at the age of forty-three and the other after an appendicectomy at the age of forty-nine. Alice was following in her mother's footsteps as far as osteoporosis was concerned, and by the age of fifty-eight had developed an obvious hump on her back. X-rays revealed several crushed spinal vertebrae in her thoracic spine, and her bone density values were very low and getting worse every year. Alice knew she needed oestrogen, but she was afraid to take it because she feared that it would cause a recurrence of her blood clots. I persuaded Alice to try the oestrogen patch and she began using it regularly. She was greatly relieved to be able to take a form of oestrogen that was safe and effective, and we both relaxed six months later, when tests showed that she had stopped losing calcium from her spine.

The oestrogen patch can be a godsend to women unable to tolerate oestrogen implants or tablets. It is also better for high-risk women, such as those with liver disorders, high blood pressure, varicose veins, or a history of thrombosis, and for those who cannot stop smoking. The patch is useful as well for women with bowel problems, such as Crohn's disease, ulcerative colitis, irritable bowel syndrome, and poor intestinal absorption, as these conditions may cause hormone tablets to be poorly absorbed.

VAGINAL OESTROGEN

Oestrogen can also be taken via the vagina. Indeed, this is a very popular form of HRT. It is particularly useful if you have a lot of vaginal dryness or shrinkage; it will also reduce bladder problems such as urinary frequency, incontinence, or a burning sensation with urination. Oestrogen cream is easily inserted with a vaginal applicator, which enables you to place the cream high into the vagina (see Figure 13). It is best done last thing at night before going to bed, after sexual intercourse, and after emptying the bladder. Oestrogen is rapidly absorbed through the vaginal lining into the bloodstream, and reasonable levels of blood oestrogen can be achieved.

Uterus

Cervix

Applicator

Pessary cream

Figure 13 **Application of vaginal cream**

Generally, vaginal oestrogen cream is prescribed for once-a-week use, but you may use it more often if you desire. If you still have your uterus, the regular, frequent use of vaginal oestrogen should be accompanied by a twelve-day course of progesterone tablets every two or three months to guard against oestrogenic over-stimulation of the uterus. These progesterone tablets may bring on a light menstrual period.

Some women find the vaginal oestrogens are satisfactory and do not take any other forms of oestrogen. Several women have told me that they feel very sexy several hours after using these creams! Others find the creams a little messy and prefer to use vaginal oestrogen suppositories, which are inserted high into the vagina with an applicator. Regular oestrogen tablets can also be inserted into the vagina. If they are placed high enough in the vagina, they are well absorbed. One brand, called Vagifem, comes with an easy-to-use vaginal applicator. If you find that taking oestrogen tablets orally is causing side-effects such as nausea or fluid retention, you may find that changing to the vaginal route of administration will eliminate these side-effects.

Oestrogen is also available in the form of a ring-shaped pessary under the brand name Estring that enables oestrogen to be absorbed for a three month period before it needs to be replaced. The ring sits high up in the vagina in much the same way as a vaginal diaphragm and the oestrogen it contains is gradually absorbed through the walls of the vagina.

HORMONE IMPLANTS

Hormone implants are small, solid pellets of natural hormones that resemble tiny pieces of spaghetti. They are implanted (inserted) into the fatty layer under the skin of the abdomen or buttocks. A doctor uses a local anaesthetic and a small hollow tube with a sharp cutting edge to slide the pellet neatly into the fatty tissue (see Figure 14). This procedure should not be painful. The implants release hormones slowly and directly into the bloodstream for six to twelve months, depending on the dosage; this is great for those who cannot remember to take tablets.

Implants of natural oestrogen (oestradiol) and testosterone have been used for many years in Europe, South Africa, and Australia, where they are becoming increasingly popular. However, hormone implants should be inserted only by doctors who have special expertise in this area. This is because if they produce unwanted side-effects, removal of the implants can be difficult.

Of all the types of HRT, an implant comes closest to copying the function of your own ovaries, as in both cases oestrogen is released directly into the bloodstream and is carried to the various oestrogen-dependent tissues of your body. This means your hungry cells can get their supply of precious oestrogen before the liver cells can break it down. Unfortunately, this is not so with oestrogen tablets which are first broken down during passage through the liver after their absorption from the gut. Thus the liver could be said to weaken the effect of oestrogen tablets upon your cells, whereas the oestrogen implant is able to deliver an unweakened supply of oestrogen.

Figure 14

Implants are particularly good for menopausal women with severe symptoms and/or symptoms that do not respond to other treatment. It is definitely true that for a small percentage of women, no other type of HRT works as well as hormone implants. I have found this to be more likely in the following cases: after hysterectomy (surgical removal of the uterus); after oophorectomy (surgical removal of the ovaries), especially in younger women; and in premature menopause.

Janet, aged fifty-six, was having a stressful menopause despite taking oestrogen and progesterone tablets regularly. Her hot flushes and sweats made her feel dirty, her clothes clung to her flesh and she felt as though ants were crawling under her skin. Her libido had vanished and a deep depression had set in. Janet was told that these symptoms were all in her mind and that she needed a good psychiatrist. A blood test revealed low levels of oestradiol and testosterone and we agreed that she should have an oestrogen and testosterone implant. Three weeks later her blood test showed normal levels of oestrogen and testosterone and Janet was relieved of the symptoms that were supposedly 'all in her mind'.

Some of the world's foremost experts on the menopause use hormone implants as first-line therapy in menopausal women who complain of fatigue, depression or loss of libido.[3] Oestradiol implants have been shown to increase bone density and can be used to prevent osteoporosis. Psychological and sexual problems occurring after the menopause may be greatly helped by taking the male hormone testosterone; generally it is only necessary for a few months. Testosterone does not work well in tablet form and an implant or intra-muscular injection of natural testosterone provides an ideal alternative.[4] Testosterone implants and/or injections generally produce a feeling of mental, physical and sexual well-being and most women are very happy with their effects. It is only fair to warn any woman considering a testosterone implant that it may cause a slight increase in facial hair or pimples, but this decreases when the dose of testosterone is reduced or left off in subsequent implants of oestrogen. If the dose of testosterone implant is kept at 50 mg every six to twelve months, it is highly unlikely that undesirable side-effects such as facial hair, acne, voice changes or increased cholesterol will occur.

It is important that your suitability for and dosage of oestrogen implant is carefully considered as, once inserted, the implants are difficult to remove if overdose or side-effects occur. Side-effects are mostly confined to tender breasts or an increase in the heaviness of menstrual bleeding but the latter can usually be controlled by increasing the dosage of progesterone.

For some women (around 3–8 per cent), the implants may be effective only temporarily. Such women find themselves requiring implants at increasingly shorter intervals, even though their blood tests show very high levels of oestrogen. This type of addictive reaction is called tachyphylaxis, in which it seems as if a woman simply cannot get enough oestrogen. This is not good, as it is unnatural for the body continually to have very high levels of oestrogen, mainly because it theoretically increases the risk of breast or uterine cancer. Women who become 'addicted' to high levels of oestrogen should be switched to smaller-dose oestrogen patches. They can also benefit greatly from taking a number of nutritional and dietary supplements every day, including 4 grams of evening primrose oil, 200 milligrams of vitamin B6, a balanced vitamin B complex, and antioxidants: 1,000 milligrams of vitamin C, 20 milligrams of beta-carotene, 500 international units of vitamin E, and 50 micrograms of selenium. This is because very high levels of oestrogen may lead to nutritional deficiencies and imbalances in the body. A safe and reasonable level of oestrogen in the body is 300–500 pmol/L, as determined by a blood test.

Towards the end of the life of your implant you should have a blood test to check your oestrogen and follicle-stimulating hormone (FSH) levels so that another implant can be inserted before oestrogen deficiency returns.

As you can see, there are many different ways you can take hormone replacement. What works for one woman does not necessarily work for another, and time and patience may be needed to find out the correct dosages and form of HRT for you, tailor-made to keep your feeling well and to stabilize your blood levels of hormones in the normal range.

CHAPTER FIVE

THE MOST-ASKED QUESTIONS ABOUT MENOPAUSE

Many women are confused about important aspects of menopause, and find it difficult to get direct and clear answers. When it comes to menopause, ignorance is not bliss. It can be frightening to feel that your body is going through incomprehensible changes over which you have no control.

Each section in this chapter is devoted to one of the questions my women patients ask me most often. It is designed to give you accurate answers and vital information that will enable you to make informed decisions. It will help to demystify menopause and put you back in control of your life and your health.

WHEN WILL I GO THROUGH MENOPAUSE?

The average age at menopause is fifty years. However, some women go through a premature menopause in their twenties or thirties, while others continue to menstruate up until their late fifties.

There are a number of factors that are known to influence the age at which a woman experiences menopause. If you started menstruating early in life (before ten years of age), you are more likely to have a late menopause. A woman who has had a hysterectomy, even if she has kept her ovaries, may experience menopause up to four years earlier than average. This is because the blood supply to the ovaries may be decreased after removal of the uterus. Other factors associated with early menopause include smoking, radiation exposure, and chemotherapy. Menopause can also be brought on artificially if the ovaries are removed through surgery or if they are treated with radiation therapy.

How Long Does Menopause Last?

The word menopause means the cessation of menstrual bleeding – that is, the last menstrual period. However, in the period before, during, and after the last period, huge hormonal changes, such as large and sometimes rapid fluctuations in the levels of sex hormones, take place in the body. This period of time is called the perimenopause or the climacteric. Common symptoms are hot flushes, sweating, changes in menstrual bleeding, and mood changes. These symptoms may last for a variable period of time, and the variation among individual women is quite amazing. Some women find that perimenopause lasts only a few months, while others find that it lasts for ten to fifteen years. Thankfully, with appropriate HRT and/or natural therapies, you can avoid the unpleasant symptoms of this time altogether!

After the perimenopausal period, a woman becomes postmenopausal, with very low and stable levels of sex hormones in her body (unless, of course, she is taking hormone replacement therapy).

Should I Take Hormones?

When you look at the advantages and powerful influences of hormone replacement therapy, it is tempting to believe that all women should take oestrogen for menopause. It can effectively relieve acute menopausal discomforts, such as hot flushes and flagging libido, and also dramatically reduces the risk of osteoporosis and cardiovascular disease. But each woman is unique. Some women have no symptoms and are not at risk of developing cardiovascular disease or osteoporosis, so there is no medical reason for them to take HRT. But every menopausal woman has the right to be examined and tested. And if you are found to be at risk of developing one of these serious health problems, or if you are suffering from unpleasant menopausal symptoms, you should be offered the option of taking HRT. Furthermore, there are many popular misconceptions about HRT (for a look at some of the more common ones, see Hormonal Myths, page 97). Consequently, all women should receive complete and accurate information about HRT before deciding whether or not to try it.

IF I TAKE HRT, HOW LONG WILL I NEED IT?

Around 40 per cent of women still complain of symptoms due to oestrogen deficiency ten years after the start of menopause. They may still be troubled by hot flushes, vaginal dryness, sweating, and loss of sexual desire and enjoyment. Such symptoms last for different periods of time in different people, so the appropriate duration of oestrogen replacement therapy for the control of acute menopausal symptoms varies, depending on what an individual woman needs.

To prevent osteoporosis, oestrogen replacement therapy must be taken for a period of fifteen to twenty years. Taking oestrogen protects your bones against calcium loss and your heart and blood vessels against disease, but this protection ceases once oestrogen therapy is stopped. Many doctors therefore believe that women at risk of developing osteoporosis should stay on oestrogen for life, provided they feel well and receive regular medical check-ups. Furthermore, it is never too late to begin HRT. Some women can still benefit if they start it in their sixties or seventies.

We know that fewer than one-third of postmenopausal women continue with HRT over the long term. This is because many women feel uncomfortable about making a long-term commitment to HRT, as there is continuing controversy as to whether it may cause an increased risk of breast cancer or liver disease. I believe that the duration of HRT is a very individual matter that needs to be reviewed regularly throughout the postmenopausal period. Ultimately, the length of time you take HRT should be your informed choice. You will need to read all of this book and communicate with your doctor before you decide what is right for you.

What If I Get Side-effects?

Usually, side-effects from HRT are minor and can be overcome by trying smaller doses of hormones or taking a different form of HRT. Rarely, high doses of the oral forms of HRT can cause thrombosis (the formation of a blood clot or clots in the blood vessels), and this may produce pain and swelling in the legs. HRT may cause migraine headaches in women who are predisposed to them, and the migraines can be preceded by disturbances in vision or speech or by a sensation of weakness in the limbs. This is not common, but if it occurs you should immediately cease taking HRT and consult your doctor. Women more prone to such side-effects are those who smoke, who are obese, or who have high blood pressure, varicose veins, or a past history of blood clots or strokes. For such high-risk women, oestrogen patches are much safer than other forms of HRT.

Some women on HRT complain of a mild to moderate weight gain. This is because HRT may cause a slight increase in appetite and fluid retention. Weight gain can be avoided by reducing the dose of HRT, avoiding strong androgenic (masculinizing) progestogens such as norgestrel and norethisterone, reducing the amount of saturated fat in the diet, and getting regular exercise.

Fewer than 50 per cent of women who start on HRT continue with treatment for more than a few months. Yet to prevent osteoporosis, HRT must be taken for fifteen to twenty years, if not for life. The reason many women give up on HRT is that they get annoying side-effects. I have designed a table to help you and your doctor work out some practical solutions and alternatives if you run into problems with HRT (see Table 5). Remember, patience is a virtue!

Side-effects can be minimized by starting with small doses of natural hormones and, if necessary, gradually increasing the dose

HORMONAL MYTHS

Many women are reluctant to consider hormone replacement therapy because of some of the things they may have heard about it. But many of these things are really nothing more than hormonal myths. The following table lists some of these common misconceptions as well as the actual facts about HRT.

MYTH	TRUTH
If I start on HRT, I'll never be able to come off it.	Not true. HRT is not addictive.
Menopausal problems can always be fully treated with nutritional medicine.	Each woman is an individual. Some require oestrogen replacement therapy for optimum health and well-being.
HRT should always be taken in the lowest possible dose for the shortest possible time.	Dosage needs vary with the individual. Some women should take HRT for at least fifteen to twenty years.
HRT never causes weight gain.	HRT can cause weight gain in some women, even if they do not eat more or exercise less (see page 101).
HRT increases the risk of cancer	Properly balanced natural HRT actually reduces the risk of endometrial and ovarian cancer. In some cases it may increase the risk of breast cancer, although further long-term studies are required to confirm this. It appears to have little or no effect on other types of cancer.
If HRT brings back my periods, I might get pregnant.	This is impossible. A menopausal woman has no eggs left in her ovaries, and without eggs, conception cannot occur.
I will not need HRT until after my menstrual bleeding ceases.	Not necessarily. A deficiency of oestrogen may occur several years before this.
Menopause is a short-lived condition.	Menopause is an epoch with effects lasting until the end of life.

until you feel relieved of your symptoms. Your doctor may need to adjust your dosage and method of taking HRT several times to find a programme that suits you as an individual and avoids annoying side-effects.

WON'T HRT MAKE ME GAIN WEIGHT?

In my experience, approximately one in three women who start hormone replacement therapy at menopause gains a significant amount of weight. This is usually in the range of four to five pounds, but it can occasionally be much more. This tendency can be avoided by asking your doctor to prescribe natural forms of oestrogen and progesterone instead of the synthetic types of these hormones. Quite a few menopausal women find that they need to reduce the dosage of hormone replacement therapy or, if they fail, take hormone replacement therapy in the form of oestrogen patches instead of tablets to avoid gaining weight.

Oestrogen patches are sold under the brand names Estraderm, Evorel, Fematrix, Menorest, Femseven and Progynova TS and come in various strengths: 25, 37.5, 40, 50, 75, 80 and 100 micrograms. The smaller dose of oestrogen in the weaker oestrogen patches – Estraderm 25 or Evorel 25 – is most unlikely to cause weight gain. Generally speaking, it is possible, by juggling and/or reducing the doses of oestrogen and progesterone in your hormone replacement therapy, to avoid any significant weight gain.

Heavier women usually require smaller doses of hormone replacement therapy than thin women do. They may need to take smaller amounts of progesterone, either by breaking the tablets in half or quarters, or by taking them for a shorter time each calendar

TABLE 5 PROBLEM SIDE-EFFECTS OF HRT AND SUGGESTED SOLUTIONS

Many women who try hormone replacement therapy discontinue it because they are bothered by side-effects such as weight gain, headaches, or fluid retention. Yet in many cases, side-effects can be minimized or even eliminated by making adjustments in dosage or method of administration. The table below lists some of the most commonly cited troublesome side-effects of HRT and suggested solutions for them. However, you should never make any changes in your HRT programme without first consulting your doctor.

SIDE-EFFECT	SUGGESTED SOLUTION
Breast swelling and tenderness, heavy menstrual bleeding, menstrual cramps.	Breast tenderness and heavy menstrual bleeding can be caused by too much oestrogen. Reduce the dosage of oestrogen and possibly increase the dosage of progestogen. Take 3,000 mg of evening primrose oil and 50 mg of vitamin B6 daily.
Increased blood pressure, fluid retention, bloating, weight gain, aching legs.	Fluid retention can be caused by too much oestrogen. Reduce the dosage of oestrogen or change to a non-oral form such as patches. Reduce the dosage of protestogen.
Migraine headaches, nausea, vomiting.	Nausea and headaches can be caused by too much oestrogen. Change to a non-oral form of oestrogen such as patches. Begin with low-dose oestrogen patches.
Inability to tolerate menstrual bleeding.	Take both oestrogen and progestogen continuously, every day. Or consider endometrial ablation (see page 105).

SIDE-EFFECT	SUGGESTED SOLUTION
Depression, irritability, mood changes, loss of sex drive.	Change to a non-oral form of oestrogen such as injections (not available in Britain) or patches. The addition of testosterone injections or implants may be necessary, often for three to twelve months only. Change to a natural progesterone (e.g. suppositories or lozenges).
Chloasma (dark and/or blotchy brown facial pigmentation).	Reduce the dosage of oestrogen and change to oestrogen patches. Avoid exposure to sunlight; wear a hat and sun-block when outdoors.
Premenstrual symptoms such as depression and/or irritability during progestogen therapy.	Depression and symptoms of premenstrual syndrome can be caused by too much progestogen. Reduce the dosage of progestogen (to 2.5 milligrams of Provera daily, for example), or change to natural progesterone tablets, suppositories, or injections. Natural progesterone is less likely to cause mood disorders than synthetic progestogens are. Take progesterone less often, every two or three months instead of every month. Take 50 milligrams of vitamin B6 and 3,000 milligrams of evening primrose oil daily.
Oestrogen deficiency symptoms while on HRT.	See the Oestrogen Level Score Chart on page 21. Have a blood test to check your blood level of oestradiol. If it is on the low side, increase the dosage of oral oestrogen or add or change to oestrogen patches or injections. For vaginal dryness, add oestrogen cream.
Development of large varicose veins or worsening of existing varicose veins.	Reduce the dosage of oestrogen or change to oestrogen patches. Take 500 IU of vitamin E daily.

month. Natural progesterone tablets are unlikely to cause any big gains in weight and may be preferred by women with weight problems.

If, despite all these measures, hormone replacement therapy still causes unwanted weight gain, you may decide to give up HRT altogether, but check with your doctor first. You may be losing the great advantages that oestrogen replacement therapy offers your skeleton and blood vessels. You may also benefit from specific changes in diet tailored to your individual metabolism (see Body Types and HRT, below).

If after all consideration you do decide to give up on hormone replacement therapy, I suggest that you consume plenty of foods that are high in calcium, vitamin D, and natural plant oestrogens. Natural plant oestrogens can be found in many foods, such as green beans and soya-beans. Further information about foods that are high in natural plant oestrogens and calcium may be found in Chapter 6.

BODY TYPES AND HRT

Weight gain is a not uncommon side-effect of hormone replacement therapy. However, the exact way in which you may be affected depends on your body type. Generally speaking, all women fall into four different body type categories – android, gynaecoid, lymphatic, and thyroid (see illustrations). You can be a combination of two of these four different types, but most women are predominantly one type or another.

The android type is characterized by a strong, sometimes thickset skeletal frame, broad shoulders, a wide ribcage, and muscular limbs. The waist is not well defined and the pelvic bones are narrow, so that the physique is relatively straight up and down. There is a lack of feminine curves and the figure is somewhat 'boyish'. The buttocks and thighs are muscular and the pelvis and buttocks do not curve outwards below a somewhat thick waist. The android-type woman's limb bones are large, and she has more muscle mass and less fat tissue than the other body types. If excess weight gain occurs, fat is deposited in the upper part of the body, above the pelvis. This results in a thickening of the 'apple-shaped obesity'. An android-type woman, if taking excessive or unnecessary HRT, will put on weight in the upper portion of her body, especially if she is taking excessive progesterone or testosterone.

The gynaecoid type is characterized by a pear shape, with the buttocks and thighs flowing outwards below a narrow waist. The buttocks are curved and rounded, and the thighs curve out to the sides. The shoulders are small to average in breadth; the waist is tapered and much smaller than the hips; and the pelvis is wide. The bones of the limbs are slender, with tapered, fine forearms, wrist, shins, and ankles. If weight gain occurs, fat is deposited first on the buttocks, thighs, and breasts, and later over the lower abdomen in front of the pubic bones, while the forearms and shins remain relatively slim. The bottom has a tendency to droop downward over the backs of the thighs if weight gain occurs. A gynaecoid-type woman who takes excessive or unnecessary HRT will put on weight primarily in the pelvic area, buttocks, and thighs. This type of woman becomes more pear-shaped as she gains weight.

The lymphatic type is characterized by a generalized thickening and puffiness of the tissues underlying the skin. This is because she retains lymphatic fluid and fat, especially in her limbs, which gives her thick arms and legs, with a straight up and down look along their length. The ankles and wrists are thick and puffy in appearance. The shoulders, breasts, and ribcage are average in size, and the abdomen may protrude in front. The torso, like the limbs, is relatively straight up and down, with a thick waist and moderate curves outward on the buttocks and thighs. The bones and the muscles are average in

Android body shape
left: overweight, right: ideal weight

Gynaecoid body shape
left: overweight, right: ideal weight

Lymphatic body shape
left: overweight, right: ideal weight

Thyroid body shape
left: overweight, right: ideal weight

size and their shape is not clearly defined. If a lymphatic-type woman gains excessive weight, the extra fat will be distributed all over her body – in the legs, feet, arms, hands, buttocks, abdomen, trunk, neck, and face. Lymphatic-type women gain weight very easily and have often been chubby since childhood. If a lymphatic-type woman takes excessive or unnecessary HRT, she will put on weight all over, in the form of an extra layer of fat over the entire body. She will also retain fluid in her limbs.

The thyroid type is characterized by a narrow streamlined shape, with fine bones and long limbs. Many thyroid-type women are tall, but even those who are not give the impression of being taller than they are, because of their relatively long legs and arms. They have narrow waists and small curves outwards on the buttocks and thighs. Their fingers, toes, and necks are long and narrow, like their limbs. Their bones are fine and the bone structure is clearly defined, with the ribs and bony protuberances (knobs) around the joints being very evident. If weight gain occurs, fat is deposited around the abdomen and upper thighs, while the upper part of the body and limbs remain slim. Thyroid-type women gain weight less easily than the other body shapes. Generally speaking, the thin thyroid types tolerate higher doses of HRT without significant weight gain.

If you have worked with your doctor to find the correct dose of HRT and you still find yourself gaining weight and don't know why, investigate your diet more thoroughly. You may be consuming excess calories or a diet that is wrong for your particular body shape. In my experience, each of the four body shapes has a different metabolism and hormonal balance, and you will lose weight most effectively if you follow a scientifically balanced diet and eat combinations of food that are right for your body shape. This unique weight-loss approach is called the Body-Shaping Diet. A full discussion of this approach is available in my book, *The Body-Shaping Diet*, which gives step-by-step meal plans and recipes formulated for each of the four body shapes to achieve effective weight loss and body shaping.[1]

IS THERE ANY WAY TO AVOID BLEEDING ON HRT?

Some postmenopausal women cannot cope with any bleeding, even if it is regular and predictable, at an age in life when they wish to be free of periods, tampons, and inconvenient napkins and pads. If you feel like this, tell your doctor. He or she can prescribe progestogen tablets to be taken every day along with your oestrogen therapy. This will usually prevent any bleeding after three to four months of continual therapy.

Some women prefer to work with their doctors to try to manipulate the doses of HRT to reduce the amount and/or frequency of bleeding. This can be done by taking the progestogen course once every two or three months, instead of monthly, by increasing the strength of the progestogen tablet, or by reducing the amount of oestrogen.

A new surgical technique is now available that enables a surgeon to remove the endometrium (the lining of the uterus) while leaving the uterine walls intact. This is called *endometrial ablation*. In this procedure, the surgeon destroys the bleeding surface of the uterus with high-frequency radio waves or laser beams. Endometrial ablation can be done using a hysteroscope inserted through the cervix, so that no incision or stitches are required. This reduces the amount of pain, post-operative discomfort, and time off work the procedure entails. Since it is performed under general anaesthesia, endometrial ablation is a hospital procedure, but it is usually considered outpatient surgery (no overnight hospital stay is required).

The success of endometrial ablation varies. Afterwards, you

may find that you have no further bleeding or that the amount of bleeding is reduced to some degree. The amount of this reduction varies from woman to woman. For the best results, go to a gynaecologist who has a lot of experience in performing hysteroscopy and endometrial ablation. After an endometrial ablation, it is still necessary to take some progesterone tablets every month (because you still have your uterus), but your menstrual bleeding will be much less or even nonexistent.

Some women become so annoyed and fatigued by the bleeding HRT produces that they consider the option of hysterectomy. This is because a woman without a uterus can take oestrogen by itself without any progestogen and have no bleeding at all. A hysterectomy, however, is major surgery, and should be considered only when other measures, such as changes in the HRT regimen or endometrial ablation, offer no relief.

ARE THERE ANY REASONS WHY I SHOULDN'T TAKE OESTROGEN?

Modern-day natural HRT is very flexible and safe, and only a minority of women are told by their doctors that they should avoid it. However, if you suffer from or have a history of any of the following problems, you will probably be advised never to take oestrogen:

● Oestrogen-sensitive cancer, such as breast or endometrial cancer. Doctors generally are reluctant to give oestrogen to women who have previously been treated for uterine cancer, because it is possible that oestrogen may stimulate the distant spread of the cancer. However, if the cancer was detected in the early stages and was determined to be of a less aggressive type, and if the patient has remained cancer-free for at least two years, some doctors feel it is safe to prescribe oestrogen in small doses if a patient complains of severe symptoms of oestrogen deficiency. Some women who have been successfully treated for breast cancer find that they are unable to tolerate a complete lack of sex hormones in their bodies, and HRT programmes using very small doses of oestrogen and larger doses of progesterone can often be worked out for them. They may choose to take this type of HRT after weighing all the pros and cons with a cancer specialist. If the cancer has been completely removed and there is no sign of invasion into the local blood vessels, and the lymph glands in the armpits are free of cancer, there is roughly a 75 per cent chance of a complete cure, and as far as we know, taking HRT does not dramatically change this. A woman may live another twenty to thirty years after successful treatment for breast cancer, and she may not want to run the increased risk of bone fracture or heart attack that can occur without oestrogen.

- Severe liver disease, such as cirrhosis. Severe liver disease makes it difficult for your liver to break down or metabolize oestrogen. Normal doses of oestrogen replacement usually overtax a diseased liver so that liver function may worsen. Mild to moderate liver disease is not necessarily a contra-indication to oestrogen replacement, although in such a case I would advise that you use only oestrogen patches or vaginal oestrogen, as these are most unlikely to overtax your liver. It is best to avoid oral oestrogens in all cases of liver disease. If you have liver disease, you will need to ask your gastroenterologist about the type of liver disease you have. Liver function is easily checked with a blood test.

There are several other medical problems that make many doctors very cautious about prescribing oestrogen. They are not, however, absolute reasons why you cannot take HRT; you can, but extra vigilance and care are required. These medical problems are:

- Recent or severe blood clots or thrombosis. The statistical risk of blood clots is not increased by HRT, but if there is a past history of clots, many doctors prefer to use the oestrogen patches, as they are the safest way of taking HRT.

● Mild liver disease (see above).

● Severe high blood pressure that is difficult to control with drugs.

● Fibroids or endometriosis. With HRT, pain and irregular bleeding can be a problem and surgical treatment may be required.

● Gall bladder disease problems may be aggravated by HRT.

● Benign breast disease (mastopathy, fibrocystic disease of the breast, or chronic cystic mastitis). This may be aggravated by HRT.

● Systemic lupus erythematosus. Lupus may be aggravated by HRT.

If you are suffering from symptoms of oestrogen deficiency but feel that oestrogen replacement therapy is too dangerous for you, I recommend that you increase the amount of foods in your diet that are sources of natural plant oestrogens (see Chapter 6).

WILL HRT INCREASE MY RISK OF CANCER?

If all the published literature and clinical trials to date are analysed, it can be concluded that, generally speaking, death rates from all cancers are not increased by the correct use of HRT. However, very long-term studies are not yet available. It will be several decades before the real effect of natural HRT in promoting or reducing different types of cancer will be known. The following reflect the current state of medical knowledge regarding the effect of HRT on the incidence of different types of cancer.

ENDOMETRIAL AND OVARIAN CANCER

Modern combination HRT appears to reduce the risk of endometrial cancer, as well as that of ovarian cancer, perhaps by as much as 40 per cent. This applies only if progesterone is taken for at least ten to fourteen days out of every monthly cycle. If only oestrogen is taken, there is an increased risk of cancer of the uterus. This is why a woman who has a uterus must take progesterone in addition to oestrogen. A woman taking combination HRT actually has less risk of developing uterine cancer than a woman who is not on HRT.

BREAST CANCER

Many women are reluctant to take HRT because they fear that it will increase their chances of developing breast cancer. This remains a complicated and controversial issue, especially as we are talking about the most common cancer in Western women. Statistics show that breast cancer affects one in every thirteen women by the age of seventy-five and one in eight women who have a family history of this disease (a mother or sister who has had breast cancer). In some cancerous tumours, a substance called oestrogen-receptor protein is present, which increases the possibility that the cancer may be promoted by oestrogen therapy.

The incidence of breast cancer continues to rise progressively throughout life, so one certainly would not want to do anything during midlife that might further increase this risk. Women who are most at risk of developing breast cancer include those who have never given birth or who were over thirty when they had their first child, obese women, women who went through puberty early (before the age of eleven) and/or went through menopause late (after the age of fifty-four), and those with a family history of breast cancer. A common feature among these factors is a prolonged and constant exposure to oestrogen from the ovaries. Women who eat diets high in fat and low in fibre have higher blood levels of oestrogen than women on low-fat, high-fibre diets, and they also have a much higher incidence of breast cancer, so it seems that we have yet another possible link between oestrogen and breast cancer.

Notwithstanding these theoretical considerations, however, of nearly thirty studies examining the relationship between oestrogen replacement and breast cancer, the majority have failed to indicate a definitive for or against.[2] Individually, these studies have found either a small decrease or a small increase in the incidence of breast cancer in users of HRT. A widely publicized 1989 Swedish study linked oestrogen with a slightly increased risk of breast cancer after six or more years of use. However, the conclusions were premature, as the researchers followed up on participants for an average duration of only 5.7 years, yet it is known that most breast cancers take seven years to grow large enough to be detected. Further, the same study found that when women using oestrogen developed breast cancer, their survival rate was significantly better than that of women not on oestrogen.

A very useful overview of twenty-three studies suggests that HRT neither increases nor decreases the incidence of breast cancer.[3] However, the results of studies on long-term (more than ten years) use of HRT counteract this finding and suggest that there may be a significant increase in the risk of breast cancer. This increase is in the order of 1.3, which means that if you take oestrogen replacement therapy for more than ten years, you may have a 30 per cent increased risk of breast cancer.[4] Although the studies that show this increased risk are only population studies that surveyed women on HRT, rather than rigorously designed scientific trials comparing the experience of a group of women taking HRT with that of a group taking a placebo, they still should make a doctor cautious about prescribing high or prolonged doses of oestrogen replacement therapy to a woman with a known high risk of breast cancer. In such a case, if oestrogen therapy is necessary, I believe it is wise to use smaller or intermittent doses of oestrogen replacement therapy. Long-term studies have also found that the risk of breast cancer does not increase until after five years of oestrogen replacement therapy. This is reassuring for women who want to take oestrogen replacement therapy for only a short time.[5]

In summary, with HRT of less than five years' duration, there is probably no increase in the incidence of breast cancer. The incidence may increase after five years of HRT, and this increase appears to be in the range of 30 per cent. This will make many women reluctant to take long-term HRT. Furthermore, while it appears that the incidence of breast cancer may increase with long-term HRT, women who get breast cancer while on HRT are less likely to die from the disease.

A new study has found that there was an elevated risk of invasive breast cancer among postmenopausal women who were currently taking oestrogen alone or both oestrogen and progestogens.[6] The increase in risk was most pronounced among women over the age of fifty-five and was largely limited to those who had used hormone therapy for five or more years. They found that the addition of progestins to oestrogen does not reduce the risk of breast cancer. The study concluded that the significant increase in the risks of breast cancer among postmenopausal women over fifty-five who are currently taking hormones and who have used this therapy for five or more years suggests that the risks and benefits of hormone therapy among older women should be carefully assessed.

SKIN CANCER

Studies suggest that the use of oestrogen has no adverse effect on the subsequent development of malignant melanoma or other skin cancers. These cancers are primarily related to exposure to the sun's ultraviolet rays, rather than to hormonal factors.

In summary, it does not appear that properly balanced, natural HRT substantially increases the incidence of any cancers, apart from breast cancer. Moreover, the slight increase in the death rate from cancer is small compared to the reduction in the death rate from osteoporosis, heart disease, and stroke in oestrogen users. Of course, statistics are a generalization, and an individual woman may not wish to base her personal decision about HRT on the results of large population groups. In the final analysis, it is important that you feel good about your own decision regarding HRT. You need to trust your own instincts and judgement and those of your own doctor.

WHAT SHOULD I DO IF I HAVE IRREGULAR BLEEDING?

In a woman taking HRT, it is normal for vaginal bleeding to occur within a few days of stopping the progestogen tablets. If bleeding starts while you are still taking the progestogen tablets, consult your doctor. It may be necessary to change the dose or type of progestogen tablets.

If bleeding occurs at any other time of the cycle, particularly when you are not taking your progestogen tablets, it can be a sign of a health problem such as a uterine polyp, uterine infection, fibroids, or uterine cancer. If you experience this type of abnormal irregular bleeding, you should see your gynaecologist, who will undertake investigations to find the cause of bleeding. Similarly, if you are postmenopausal (that is, if you have not had regular menstrual periods for twelve months) and are not taking replacement hormones, you should consult your gynaecologist about any bleeding from the vagina. The gynaecologist will need to take samples of cells from the entire surface of the endometrium (the inner lining of the uterus) for testing, so that no areas are missed. To do this, your gynaecologist may do a curettage or a hysteroscopy with directed endometrial biopsies. (For information about these procedures, see Chapter 3.) With the hysteroscope, abnormal areas of the uterus can easily be seen, then biopsied (sampled) with a curette and sent to a laboratory for testing. Once this has been done, you will know whether or not your irregular bleeding is a sign of disease, and necessary treatment, if any, can be begun. If your tests show that all is well, you may start or continue taking HRT if you wish.

WILL I BECOME LESS FEMININE AFTER MENOPAUSE?

The menopausal ovary produces very little oestrogen but continues to make androgens, the so-called 'male' sex hormones, which promote the development of masculine characteristics. This may cause a hormonal imbalance in which a menopausal woman has a relative excess of masculinizing hormones. In some women, this may result in an increase in the amount of facial hair, thinning of the scalp hair, coarsening of the skin and facial features, shrinkage of the breasts, and a slight deepening of the voice. This is not inevitable, however, and there are measures you can take to combat these unpleasant symptoms. (See What Can I Do if I Have Too Many Male Hormones? on page 116 for a summary of available strategies.)

In most cases, such hormonal imbalances can easily be fixed by simply taking natural oestrogen replacement. This increases the amount of feminizing hormones in your body and at the same time reduces the production of masculinizing hormones in the ovaries. This will greatly lessen the development of masculine features.

If oestrogen replacement alone is not sufficient to prevent excessive growth of facial hair or thinning of the scalp hair, it may be necessary to use a special hormone commonly called an 'anti-male hormone'. Spironolactone (also sold under the brand name Aldactone) is one variety of anti-male hormone. Many women find that spironolactone, taken either by itself or in combination with natural oestrogen, is sufficient to control excessive facial and body hair as well as acne. Spironolactone takes six to twelve months to be really effective in controlling these symptoms of excessive masculinizing hormones.

Another anti-male hormone is cyproterone acetate (sold under the brand name Androcur), which reduces the production and action of masculinizing hormones in the body. It also acts like progesterone and can be prescribed along with oestrogen to regulate and balance menstrual blood flow.

If you find unwelcome masculine changes occurring in your body but do not want to take hormonal therapy, there is no need for you to feel that you cannot look and feel feminine. Facial and body hair can be controlled with electrolysis, bleaching, waxing, and/or shaving. A body wave or permanent can make thinning scalp hair seem fuller. A good skin-care routine and the use of products such as facial peels and masks can refine and improve the complexion. Consult a good beautician, hairdresser, or skin-care specialist.

Each day as our world becomes more polluted our bodies are burdened with toxic and artificial chemicals. Would you consciously subject your skin to further chemical stress if you didn't have to? Many people do, without giving it a second thought! They slap on a synthetic moisturizer to start their day.

A choice does exist – look for natural skin-care products containing quality ingredients such as vegetable oils (avocado, apricot, almond, wheatgerm, jojoba, evening primrose oil), vitamins such as A, C, E, essential oils, essential fatty acids, herbal extracts and biological extracts to promote a healthy glowing skin.

Essential oils and herbs have been studied for thousands of years and the Egyptians were using them to enhance beauty and health for nearly 3,000 years before Christ. Their safety and benefits have been proven time and time again. Yet many synthetic chemicals used in cosmetics today are very recent discoveries and their long-term effectiveness and/or side-effects are yet to be discovered.

The day-to-day choices we make now are important for us and our planet. Next time you take the lid off your favourite beauty product, look inside. Do you see a product made from pure natural sustainable ingredients, or a chemical cocktail of doubtful consistency?

Vital Supplements for Your Skin

To have beautiful skin it is necessary to feed your skin from within. The supplements I recommend are:

Vitamin E 500 IU daily
Evening primrose oil 3,000 mg daily
Beta-carotene 10 mg daily
Organic mineral formula 1 daily

Don't forget to drink two litres of water a day and eat lots of fresh, raw fruits and vegetables. In Chapter 6, I will discuss certain foods that are natural sources of plant oestrogens. Try to eat more of these foods regularly, as these are both slimming and feminizing. By paying attention to nutrition and exercise, keeping your weight in the healthy range, and wearing attractive clothing and jewellery, you can feel and look very much like an attractive woman. Keep in mind, too, that your mental attitude is very important. A woman who is physically and mentally active and enthusiastic will be seen as feminine and attractive by herself and by others.

WHAT IF MY MENOPAUSE IS EARLY?

Premature menopause is defined as menopause that occurs before the age of forty years. Often, the cause of premature menopause – also called early ovarian failure – cannot be determined. However, factors that may play a role are heredity, stress, heavy smoking, poor diet, excessive alcohol consumption, and autoimmune diseases (diseases caused by imbalances or malfunctions in the immune system). A woman who undergoes menopause prematurely may have been born with fewer eggs in her ovaries; if they are released at the normal rate, her eggs will soon be depleted. Radiation therapy for pelvic cancer, or chemotherapy for any type of cancer, can quickly destroy a large number of eggs, leaving an insufficient number to last for very long. A severe infection of the ovaries caused by a viral illness such as mumps can also damage large numbers of eggs. In some cases the ovaries simply become dormant, and although there may be enough eggs, they refuse to respond normally to follicle-stimulating hormone and fail to produce oestrogen. This may be temporary and the ovaries may come back into action, or it may be permanent. Surgical removal of the ovaries before the age of forty will bring on a sudden and severe premature menopause if hormone replacement is not taken.

WHAT CAN I DO IF I HAVE TOO MANY 'MALE' HORMONES?

Excessive activity of masculinizing hormones in your body, especially the free male hormones (measured by a blood test called the free androgen index or FAI), testosterone, androstenedione, and dehydroepiandrosterone may produce unsightly facial or body hair, baldness, and acne. Fortunately, we have ways to control these annoying problems.

I have developed five different hormonal regiments of relieving these symptoms. Your doctor can adapt any of these to suit your particular needs:

1 For mild cases, natural oestrogen alone may be sufficient (if you have your uterus, you will also need to take progesterone).

2 If oestrogen alone is insufficient, a regimen of natural oestrogen plus 50 to 200 milligrams of spironolactone (Aldactone) daily is effective.

3 Another alternative is a regimen of natural oestrogen daily, plus 12.5 milligrams ($^1/_4$ of a 50mg tablet) to 100 milligrams of cyproterone acetate (Androcur) daily for three weeks of every month.

4 If you are unable to tolerate oestrogen, spironolactone or Androcur can be taken alone.

5 A cortisone-type drug, taken in a small dosage (0.25 milligrams of dexamethasone, for example) at night may be helpful.

There are also a number of non-hormonal strategies that can be helpful. Consult the table below to learn about your options.

PROBLEM	STRATEGIES
Excessive facial, body hair	Under the supervision of a beautician, try one or more of the following: • Waxing (but not for very coarse, thick hair). • Bleaching (for moustache). • Depilatory creams. • Shaving (contrary to popular belief, shaving does not increase hair regrowth). • Electrolysis (for small areas only). Plucking is not recommended.
Balding; hair loss on scalp	Ask your doctor to check the function of your thyroid gland (an underactive thyroid can cause hair loss). Nutritional supplements can help greatly. Take 1,000 mg of calcium, 500 mg of magnesium, and 30 mg of zinc chelate daily, as well as trace minerals such as manganese, boron, silica, iodine, iron, chromium, molybdenum. Take 3,000 mg of evening primrose oil daily. Consider having a permanent or body wave to make hair appear fuller.
Acne	Use of herbal skin peel or clay-based mask product several times weekly or as needed. Keep your skin scrupulously clean. Use only noncomedogenic (non-pore-clogging) cosmetics and skin-care products. Take 2,000 IU of vitamin A, 500 IU of vitamin E, 2,000 mg of vitamin C, and 30 mg of zinc chelate daily. Ask your doctor about a prescription of topical tretinoin (Retin-A cream), which also has anti-ageing effects.

Women who experience premature menopause, no matter what the cause, are at early and increased risk for developing cardiovascular disease and osteoporosis. To prevent these debilitating diseases, unless she has another health problems that would prohibit it, a woman who has a premature menopause should take sufficient HRT at the time of her menopause, and ideally up to the age of fifty – in some cases, even longer, especially if her bone density is low. This should give her adequate protection.

A woman who goes through premature menopause frequently experiences a wide range of negative emotions, including anger, disbelief, shock, resentment, and shame. If you are in this situation, it is important that you receive counselling from a sympathetic doctor or qualified therapist, because if you bottle up these feelings, you may find yourself feeling very depressed.

If you have a very early menopause – say, when you are under the age of thirty – you may find it difficult to relate to much of the information available about menopause, which is usually designed with fifty-year-old women in mind, and thus you may find yourself feeling increasingly isolated. However, if you can find an understanding doctor, you should be able to work through these negative feelings. It is important to understand that menopause is not synonymous with old age. If you go through menopause early, it merely means that your ovaries have exhausted their supply of eggs sooner than normal.

A premature menopause, if properly treated, will not cause you to age more quickly, or change your personality or mental ability. Indeed, to all your friends and family, you will appear just the same as before. When it comes to your sex life, adequate HRT should help you to feel and act just as sexy as ever. You may, however, need larger doses or a different form of HRT than a woman of fifty or sixty. For information about sex and menopause, see Chapter 8.

IF I HAVE A PREMATURE MENOPAUSE, CAN I HAVE CHILDREN?

Generally, by the time premature menopause is diagnosed, a woman's fertility is very low. It is often too late to restimulate ovulation successfully, even with the use of fertility drugs. However, that doesn't necessarily mean you have to give up hope of becoming a mother. Adoption is one possibility. Recently, the option of obtaining a donor egg or embryo has also become possible. Donor eggs and embryos enable women who do not have a living supply of their own eggs to have the chance of a lifetime.

Normally an egg donor is a close relative, and both the donor and the prospective mother must take part in an in vitro fertilization (IVF) programme. The donor's ovaries are hyperstimulated to produce a crop of premium eggs. The eggs are collected and then fertilized in vitro (in a test tube), usually with the recipient's partner's sperm. The resulting embryo is then implanted into the menopausal woman's uterus, which has been suitably prepared with hormone therapy. Egg and embryo donation has been fairly successful, with up to a 20–40 per cent chance of a normal pregnancy for women who become pregnant this way.

Yes, it is amazing to think that egg donation offers menopausal women of any age the possibility to become pregnant and have a baby. I wonder if in the future we will see more women in their fifties and sixties having maternal urges?

AT THE END OF THE DAY, IS HRT REALLY SAFE?

Thus far, our experience using hormone replacement therapy in large numbers of women has produced some interesting statistics. If we look at all the major studies done so far and try to be as honest as we can (if not a little pessimistic), the overall results come out in favour of HRT, as its benefits outweigh its risks. Statistically, if we took 100,000 women and gave them oestrogen replacement therapy for ten years, we would expect that 38 more of them would get breast cancer than would have otherwise; however, 366 women would be saved from stroke, heart disease, and osteoporotic fractures.[7] In other words, more lives would be saved than lost by long-term HRT. Figure 15 shows this diagrammatically.

But the idea of treating all menopausal women with HRT remains controversial, especially as this would mean treating women with no symptoms and no risk factors for osteoporosis or cardiovascular disease. It is easy to understand why many menopausal women feel confused, when controversy and disagreement exist among the medical profession. Some women feel that they don't want to be part of a generation of 'hormone guinea pigs'. Of course, 100 years from now, we will have more conclusive evidence if taking HRT saves lives – but you may not want to wait that long!

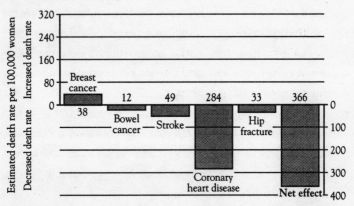

Figure 4 **Hormone replacement therapy and its relative risks**

This diagram shows the anticipated effect of HRT on the number of deaths from heart disease, osteoporosis and certain types of cancer, based on the difference in the number of deaths from these diseases in a sample of 100,000 women who took HRT for a period of ten years and that in a comparable group of women who did not take HRT.

Nothing in life can promise to be perfect. The best that today's woman can do is to seek the best compromise and balance among all her options. At the end of the day, it is you who must decide what is best for your individual lifestyle and long-term health.

Whether you decide to take HRT or not, you should see your doctor at least annually for the rest of your life, as your medical needs often change over the years. Furthermore, your risk of cancer, cardiovascular disease, and osteoporosis rises with increasing age. By visiting your doctor regularly, these degenerative diseases can be detected early and thus treated more effectively. In many cases, their progression can be prevented by regular supervision and treatment or modification of diet and lifestyle.

CHAPTER SIX

NATUROPATHIC MEDICINE FOR MENOPAUSE

For twenty years I have prescribed various combinations of vitamins, minerals, essential fatty acids, and herbs in addition to orthodox medicines to help women achieve optimum well-being during the menopausal years. The tremendous difference these nutritional supplements can make to women's health and comfort never ceases to impress me, and I firmly believe that using them is worth any extra effort and expense.

Many women prefer the process of menopause to be a natural one. The good news is that there are naturopathic means of easing many menopausal discomforts, including hot flushes, dryness and wrinkling of the skin, anxiety, and stress, as well as of improving the overall functioning of your immune system. There are also effective natural strategies for preventing or slowing the progression of some of the longer-term consequences of oestrogen deficiency, such as cardiovascular disease and osteoporosis. Even if you take hormone replacement therapy, dietary modification, nutritional and dietary supplements, herbs, and other naturopathic approaches can be used to great advantage.

NATURAL THERAPIES FOR THE SYMPTOMS OF MENOPAUSE

Many of the discomforts of the menopausal period can be helped with simple, natural treatments that you can use at home, such as increasing your consumption of foods that contain natural plant oestrogens, drinking adequate amounts of water, taking selected nutritional supplements, and using specific herbs. Table 6 gives an overview of the nutritional and dietary supplements, herbs, and other measures recommended for some of the most common menopausal symptoms. You can choose to use one, several, or all of the therapies recommended, and you can use these natural treatments either alone or in combination with hormone replacement therapy.

NATURAL PLANT OESTROGENS

Over 300 different plants contain oestrogenic substances. Although these are weak oestrogens and are present only in tiny quantities, if foods containing them are consumed regularly, they can exert a mild oestrogenic effect in humans.[1]

Alfalfa contains a plant oestrogen called coumestrol, which can actually cause infertility in animals grazing on large pastures of alfalfa grasses. Of all the plant oestrogens, coumestrol is the most potent, although it is still 200 times weaker than human oestrogens. The herb red clover also contains coumestrol and can be taken in the form of a herbal tea, or you can make fresh sprouts from red clover seeds. As some varieties of red clover are poisonous, however, it is best to obtain supplies from a reputable herbalist or health food store. Soyabeans, soyabean sprouts, and linseed meal (crushed linseeds) are excellent sources of natural oestrogens as well as of protein and essential fatty acids. They are definitely anti-ageing foods for menopausal women. For a list of foods and herbs that are good sources of plant oestrogens, see Foods Containing Natural Oestrogens, page 126.

Natural plant oestrogens provide a useful form of oestrogen supplementation for women who are unable to or who choose not to take oestrogen replacement therapy. Because these plant oestrogens are low in potency, they are safe and will not produce the side-effects sometimes seen with HRT. If you want to boost your oestrogen level, I suggest you eat approximately two cups daily of foods listed on page 126 – for example, two cups of mixed sprouts, parsley, soya beans, legumes, and fennel, along with a wide selection of fresh vegetables. Make sure you vary your sources of plant oestrogens by using different foods each day to make up your two cups' worth of oestrogenic foods.

TABLE 6

NATUROPATHIC STRATEGIES FOR MENOPAUSE

The following table offers suggestions for herbs, dietary supplements, and other natural strategies that are helpful for common menopausal symptoms. Note that the dosages for some of the items recommended are given in milligrams (mg), some in micrograms (mcg), and some in international units (IU). Both milligrams and micrograms are measures of weight (1 milligram is equal to 1,000 micrograms). International units are measures of the activity of a substance, not its weight; the number of milligrams or micrograms in an international unit therefore varies, depending on the substance being measured. Note also that appropriate doses of herbs may vary depending on the individual; if you have any doubts, consult a qualified herbalist or naturopathic physician for a personalized herbal prescription.

Some women find that taking multiple tablets of vitamins and herbs causes digestive discomfort. There are now some excellent powders containing a mixture of oestrogenic herbs, calcium, vitamins and antioxidants. These powders can be mixed in fruit juice and provide a complete nutritional formula for menopause.

PROBLEM	STRATEGIES
Hot flushes, sweating	Drink 2 litres of water daily. Take 1,000 mg of evening primrose oil and 100 IU of vitamin E, three times a day. Take one or more of the following herbs daily: • 1,000 mg of dong quai. • 500–1,000 mg of liquorice (or 1–2 cups of licorice tea). • 500–1,000 mg of black cohosh. • 500–1,000 mg of sarsaparilla (or 2–3 cups of sarsparilla tea). • 300–600 mg of chaste tree (*Vitex agnus-castus*).

Note: Liquorice can elevate blood pressure. If you have high blood presure, use it with caution or avoid it entirely.

Dry, itchy skin; vaginal dryness	Drink 2 litres of water daily. Take 1,000 mg of evening primrose oil, three times a day.

PROBLEM	STRATEGIES
Dry, itchy skin; vaginal dryness (cont.)	Take the following antioxidant supplements (with food): • 5,000 IU of vitamin A or 10 mg of beta-carotene, once daily. • 500 IU of vitamin E, once daily. • 50 mcg of selenium, once daily. • 1,000–2,000 mg of vitamin C with bioflavonoids, three times daily. Use only cold-pressed vegetable oil such as olive, linseed, grape seed, pure rape seed/canola oil, and sesame oils in cooking and salad dressings.
Fatigue, poor memory, reduced mental efficiency	Take a balanced high-potency vitamin B complex tablet or capsule daily. Take 1,000 mg of evening primrose oil, three times a day. Take 1,000 mg of ginkgo biloba, 1,000–4,000 mg of ginseng, and/or 1,000 mg of royal jelly daily.
Anxiety, irritability, mood disorders, insomnia	Take one or more of the following herbs daily (take them at bedtime for insomnia): • 250 mg of passion flower. • 1,000 mg of valerian root (or 2 cups of valerian root tea). • 1–2 cups of lime flower tea. • 1–2 tablespoons of oats. • 500 mg of skullcap. Take 4,000 mg of lecithin and 500–1,500 mg of the amino acid L-glutamine daily. Take a balanced high-potency vitamin B complex tablet or capsule daily, plus additional amount of the following: • 500 mg of vitamin B5 (pantothenic acid). • 500 mg of choline. • 10 mg of vitamin B6 (pyridoxine). • Take 500 mg of magnesium (as magnesium chelate) daily.
Muscle and joint aches and pains, degenerative diseases of the bones, joints	Take 1,000 mg of evening primrose oil, three times daily. Take 1,000 mg of fish oil daily. Take the following antioxidant supplements daily: • 10,000 IU of vitamin A or 20 mg of beta-carotene. • 2,000 mg of vitamin C (in mineral ascorbate form with muscles, and bioflavonoids). • 500 IU of vitamin E. Take the following minerals: • 1,000 mg of calcium at bedtime. • 500 mg of magnesium at bedtime.

PROBLEM	STRATEGIES
Muscle and joint aches and pains, degenerative diseases of the bones, joints (cont.)	• 1.5–3.0 mg of copper daily. • 20 mg of boron (as sodium borate) daily. • 25 mg of silica daily. • 10 mg of manganese (as manganese chelate) daily. • 30 mg of zinc (as zinc chelate) daily. Take 400 IU of vitamin D3 (cholecalciferol) and 100 mcg of vitamin K daily.
Rapid ageing of the skin, thinning hair, brittle nails, osteoporosis	Take 1,000 mg of calcium and 500 mg of magnesium at bedtime. Take the following vitamins daily: • 5,000 IU of vitamin A or 20 mg of beta-carotene. • 2,000 mg of vitamin C, preferably in mineral ascorbate form with bioflavonoids. • 500 IU of vitamin E. • 400 IU of vitamin D3 (cholecalciferol). • 100 mcg of vitamin K. Take the following trace minerals daily: • 20 mg of boron (as sodium borate). • 5 mg of copper (as copper chelate). • 30 mg of zinc (as zinc chelate). • 25 mg of silica. • 10 mg of manganese (as manganese chelate).

Plant oestrogens are also present in bourbon, whisky, gin, ouzo, and beer. These oestrogens are partly responsible for the breast development seen in alcoholic males, as their damaged livers are unable to break down and inactivate the oestrogens found in alcoholic beverages. However, I do not recommend that you try to increase your oestrogen level by drinking alcohol!

WATER

Many women find the drinking of pure water a chore and do it grudgingly, much like a penance. It is an acquired habit, but once you start drinking between one and two litres of pure water daily, your body will soon crave it if you forget. Just think how tired and sad plants look without water. Well, we are just the same!

You may flavour your water with herbal teas or a dash of fresh citrus fruit, but otherwise leave it pure, so that it can act as a cleanser and detoxifier. There is no cleanser like water. I see many women in their middle years with conditions such as joint pains, bad breath, and osteoarthritis, who did not start drinking adequate amounts of water until it was too late.

FOODS CONTAINING NATURAL OESTROGENS

A number of different foods and herbs are sources of natural plant oestrogens, and can be very helpful during menopause, the following is a list of some of the best food sources of oestrogen. These foods not only contain oestrogens, but are high in vitamins, minerals, fibre, and essential fatty acids, and they are low in saturated fat. Thus, there are many good reasons to consume them on a regular basis.

- alfalfa
- anise seed
- apples
- baker's yeast
- barley
- beets
- cabbage
- carrots
- cherries
- chickpeas
- clover
- corn
corn oil
- cowpeas (black-eyed peas)
- cucumbers

- fennel
- linseed
- garlic
- green beans
- green squash
- hops
- liquorice
- oats
- olive oil
- olives
- papaya
- parsley
- peas
- plums
- potatoes

- pumpkin
- red beans
- red clover
- rhubarb
- rice
- rye
- sage
- sesame seeds
- soyabean sprouts
- soyabeans
- split peas
- sunflower seeds •
- squash
- wheat
- yams

Start today. Drinking at least one-and-a-half litres of pure water, gradually, throughout the morning and afternoon. Keep a jug of water on your desk or carry a water bottle with you on your travels. It's well worth the extra trips to the bathroom! By drinking cool water regularly you will reduce hot flushes, headaches, joint pains, fatigue, and dry, itchy skin, and you will rejuvenate your entire cardiovascular system.

NUTRITIONAL AND DIETARY SUPPLEMENTS

There are a number of nutritional and dietary supplements that are especially useful to women who are going through menopause. In addition to supporting overall health, certain nutrients can actually help to relieve unpleasant symptoms. The supplements I recommend include vitamins, minerals, amino acids, and essential fatty acids.

Vitamin A

Vitamin A has many essential roles in the body. It is required for night vision, a healthy immune system, and reproduction. It is also an antioxidant. (For information about vitamin A's role as an antioxidant, see Chapter 7.)

Persons lacking in vitamin A may develop skin and mucous membrane disorders in which the tissues become white, hard, and chronically inflamed. This makes them more susceptible to infection.

Vitamin A comes in two forms: preformed vitamin A (retinol or retinyl esters), which is found in cod and halibut liver, cream, butter, eggs, and animal meats and livers; and provitamin A (beta-carotene), which is found in sweet potatoes, papayas, apricots, watermelons, tomatoes, and in green, yellow, and orange vegetables. The liver converts beta-carotene into vitamin A as the body needs it.

Both vitamin A and beta-carotene strengthen mucous membranes throughout the body. This is helpful for the unpleasant menopausal symptoms of vaginal dryness and fragility. I have found that the combination of vitamin A (or beta-carotene) and evening primrose oil is effective in reducing the itchy, crawling sensation in the skin that often occurs during menopause.

The recommended daily allowance of vitamin A is 1,000 micrograms (around 3,500 international units). However, smokers, regular drinkers of alcohol, junk-food consumers, diabetics, and those exposed to excessive pollutants and toxic chemicals often need more. If you have dry and irritated skin and mucous membranes, it is safe to take 10,000 international units of vitamin A or 20,000 to 25,000 international units of beta-carotene daily. Doses above 10,000 international units of vitamin A daily should not be taken without medical supervision, as very high doses (25,000 to 50,000 international units daily) can be toxic. A pregnant woman should never take more than 5,000 international units of vitamin A daily.

Unlike vitamin A, beta-carotene is non-toxic, even in high doses, so there is no need to worry about overdosage. However, no more than 25,000 international units daily is needed to achieve maximal benefits.

The B Vitamins
The B vitamins are a vital group of nutrients that are involved in the functioning of the nervous system and in maintaining healthy skin, eyes, and hair. They also support adrenal gland function and are involved in energy production. The B vitamins should always be taken as a group, in a balanced B complex supplement. If you take any of the B vitamins individually, you should also take a B complex supplement at a different time of day.

Vitamin B5 (pantothenic acid), vitamin B6 (pyridoxine), and choline are three simple and inexpensive nutrients that can neatly provide help for the common menopausal symptoms of anxiety, poor sleep, and loss of libido. Vitamin B6 is required for the conversion of amino acids into neurotransmitters (brain chemicals). In particular, B6 is essential for the conversion of the amino acid tryptophan into the neurotransmitter serotonin. Serotonin exerts an antidepressant effect, and normal amounts are required for a healthy libido. The recommended daily dose of vitamin B6 is 50 milligrams. Do not take more than this, or transient nerve damage can occur. Good food sources of vitamin B6 are meats, whole grains, and brewer's yeast.

Vitamin B5 and choline are the precursors for the neurotransmitter acetylcholine. Acetylcholine is required for the normal functioning of memory. People who suffer from anxiety often have excessive levels of adrenaline and insufficient amounts of acetylcholine in their bodies. Acetylcholine is one of the neurotransmitters required for the action of the autonomic nervous system, which is involved in sexual excitement and orgasm. Ensuring adequate levels of acetylcholine helps to maintain sexual responsiveness and enjoyment of love-making. The recommended dose of both vitamin B5 and choline is 500 milligrams daily. Vitamin B5 is present in organ meats, eggs, and whole grain cereals. Good food sources of choline include lecithin, eggs, soyabeans, cauliflower, cabbage, tofu, and tempeh.

Vitamin C
Vitamin C, or ascorbic acid, is so vital to human health that I have often thought it to be an evolutionary defect that the human body does not manufacture its own supply. Most animals produce their own supplies of vitamin C, which increase when they are under stress.

Vitamin C was made famous by the research of the late Dr Linus Pauling. Dr Pauling, twice a Nobel laureate, stated that vitamin C could prevent the common cold and treat cancer. Many doctors believe that vitamin C can reduce the severity of colds and help prevent cancer, although it cannot control established, advanced cancers. Other doctors do not believe in using nutritional supplements at all – generally because university medical schools are only just starting to include in their curricula any study of nutrition as a therapeutic tool.

Vitamin C is needed for the manufacture of collagen, which acts like a flexible or elastic protein glue in connective tissue and bone. Ensuring plentiful vitamin C helps to maintain healthy collagen, thereby keeping the skin and mucous membranes thicker and stronger and the skeleton more flexible. If your ligaments and bones are more flexible, they are less likely to be torn (sprained) or broken (fractured). Vitamin C is also a powerful antioxidant and free-radical scavenger that helps to reduce degenerative diseases and inflammation, and to slow down the ageing process. (For information about the role of vitamin C as an antioxidant, see Chapter 7.)

Vitamin C is found in high concentrations in the brain and the adrenal glands, and it is required for these organs to function under stress. I always recommend that people who are under mental or physical stress take additional vitamin C, and have found it to have a natural relaxing effect.

The recommended dose of vitamin C is quite a controversial subject among doctors. Although many agree that the UK recommended daily allowance of 30 milligrams is inadequate for optimal health, few agree with Dr Pauling that the daily requirement is between 2,000 and 9,000 milligrams. What is true is that the daily requirement for vitamin C varies greatly among individuals. Factors that increase a person's daily requirement are stress, smoking, infections, surgery, exposure to pollution, and the consumption of alcohol. If you do not eat fresh raw fruits and vegetables every day, you may be deficient in vitamin C, as the body is continually using it up. Vitamin C is destroyed by high temperatures, which is why raw foods are so important.

I believe it is imperative to get at least 1,000 milligrams daily, and if any factors that increase your need, such as those mentioned above, are present, you may require up to 6,000 milligrams daily. It is best to take it in divided doses, with food. However, it is much better to get your vitamin C from natural, fresh raw food sources than to rely on supplements alone. Good food sources of vitamin C include citrus fruits, tomatoes, capsicum, Brussels sprouts, broccoli, berries (blueberries, gooseberries, raspberries, strawberries), bananas, alfalfa, guava, potatoes, cantaloupe, sweet potatoes, spinach, watermelon, green leafy vegetables, green and red peppers, sprouted grains, and rose hips.

In most of the high-vitamin-C foods, there are also other nutrients, called bioflavonoids (or, occasionally, vitamin P). There are around 500 different bioflavonoids found in food plants. Bioflavonoids aid in the absorption and utilization of vitamin C and enhance its antioxidant properties. Some vitamin C supplements contain bioflavonoids as well.

Vitamin D

Vitamin D, or cholecalciferol, functions as both a vitamin and a hormone. Vitamin D is synthesized in the skin when the skin is exposed to the sun's ultraviolet rays. It is required for the absorption and utilization of calcium and helps calcium to be deposited in your bones. Gross deficiencies of vitamin D cause osteomalacia, which is a bone demineralizing disease not unlike osteoporosis. Osteomalacia is the adult equivalent of childhood rickets. Even marginal or slight deficiencies of vitamin D can increase your risk of osteoporosis and deterioration of the joints. Deficiencies of vitamin D can also contribute to thinning of the hair, brittleness of the nails, and rapid ageing of the skin.

Vitamin D is not present in a wide variety of foods, but is confined mainly to fish liver oils, fatty fish, liver, egg yolks, and butter, and, to a lesser degree, cows' milk. It is not unusual for women to be deficient in vitamin D, as many of us now avoid the sun; at the same time, in our constant effort to lose weight, we are reducing the amount of eggs, dairy products, and fatty fish we eat. Those who have difficulty digesting and absorbing fats can easily develop suboptimal levels of vitamin D. Your doctor can test you for vitamin D deficiency with a simple blood test.

The recommended daily allowance of vitamin D is 400 international units. Supplements of 200 to 400 international units daily are a good idea if you avoid sunlight and fatty foods. Take vitamin D supplements with meals or drink vitamin-D-fortified milk. Do not take excessive doses of vitamin D, however, as this may cause very high blood calcium levels, calcifications in the body's soft tissues and organs, and kidney stones. Doses less than 1,000 international units daily are considered most unlikely to exert any dangerous effects. Even so, if you have a tendency to develop kidney stones, you should take vitamin D or calcium supplements only under medical supervision.

Vitamin E

Vitamin E is essential for the existence of all oxygen-breathing creatures. It has a protective, or sparing, effect on oestrogen, so that your oestrogen (whether your own or from hormone replacement therapy) lasts longer. As a result, vitamin E helps to reduce hot flushes. Some women have told me that vitamin E supplements delayed menopause and the state of oestrogen deficiency. Perhaps the ancient Greeks knew of the hormonal benefits of eating foods high in vitamin E; the chemical name for vitamin E is tocopherol, which in Greek means 'to carry and bear babies'.

Together with vitamin A, vitamin E strengthens the skin and mucous membranes. Many women find that these vitamins reduce vaginal dryness and shrinkage. Vitamin E also reduces free radical damage to your cells' membranes and is a powerful anti-ageing nutrient. (For information about the actions of vitamin E as an antioxidant, see Chapter 7.)

The recommended daily dose of vitamin E is from 100 to 500 international units daily. Start slowly, gradually building up the dosage, to avoid a sudden boost to your cardiovascular system. Over the long term, daily doses of 100 international units are generally sufficient. If you find brown age spots appearing on your skin, taking additional vitamin E can reverse this degenerative process. Take 500 international units daily until the spots fade, and apply a combination of vitamin E cream and aloe vera gel to the affected areas twice daily.

Vitamin K

Vitamin K is a fat-solution vitamin that is needed for the synthesis of several blood-clotting factors, and for this reason it can reduce the heavy menstrual bleeding that is common in the perimenopausal years. Vitamin K is also needed for the mineralization of bone and helps to keep your bones stronger and more resilient to breaking. Some preliminary studies suggest that vitamin K can be significant in the prevention of osteoporosis.

Vitamin K deficiency is not common, as this nutrient is present in many different types of foods, and bacteria in the intestines synthesize a large proportion of daily vitamin K requirements. If you take antibiotics frequently, however, you can greatly reduce your production of vitamin K. A tendency to bruise easily can be a sign of vitamin K deficiency.

The recommended daily allowance for vitamin K is 65 micrograms, an amount that normally is easily obtained in the diet. Good food sources include green leafy vegetables, egg yolks, blackstrap molasses, alfalfa, kelp, nettles, dairy products, wheat bran, wheat germ, soyabean oil, and cod liver oil. Foods containing lactobacillus bacteria (such as kefir [fermented cows' milk], whey, and yoghurt) add a friendly bacterium to the intestines that produces vitamin K. If you have malabsorption or digestive problems, or take antibiotics frequently, a supplement of 50 to 100 micrograms daily is desirable.

Boron

Boron is a trace mineral found in plant foods, and its health benefits are becoming increasingly evident. A study done in 1987 found that boron may be helpful in preventing osteoporosis.[2] Twelve postmenopausal women between the ages of forty-eight and eighty-two were studied for twenty-four weeks. During the first seventeen weeks they were given a diet low in boron (which is what many women normally consume), and during the subsequent seven weeks they received 3 milligrams of boron daily.

Eight days after they began taking boron, the women's urinary losses of calcium and magnesium were greatly reduced, and they had significant increases (approximately twofold) in their production of oestrogen and testosterone. Reducing the loss of magnesium from the body is very desirable, as magnesium is essential for a healthy cardiovascular system and skeleton. This research suggests that taking boron supplements, especially if your dietary intake of boron is low, can cause favourable changes in mineral metabolism that can reduce, and may even prevent, the loss of mineral from the bones (osteoporosis). Boron is also necessary for healthy hair, skin, and nails, and an adequate intake of boron may help prevent muscle and joint aches and pains.

Foods high in boron include fruits, vegetables, and sesame seeds. Meat and poultry, on the other hand, are low in boron. Boron is available in supplement form, most commonly as sodium borate. An appropriate dosage would be 5 to 20 milligrams daily.

Calcium

As discussed in Chapter 2, many perimenopausal women do not consume the recommended daily allowance of 1,000 milligrams of calcium. This can increase their risk of developing osteoporosis, cardiovascular disease, arthritis, cramps, and fragile skin. Calcium and magnesium work together to form bone substance and to regulate muscular tone, and they are required in a ratio of 2:1 (that is, 200 milligrams of calcium per 100 milligrams of magnesium). Every woman should consume at least 1,000 milligrams of calcium per day, either from food sources or in supplement form (see page 157).

Copper

Copper is an essential trace mineral. Together with iron, copper enables the blood protein haemoglobin to carry precious oxygen to your cells.

Copper is a component in superoxide dismutase, an antioxidant enzyme produced by the body that protects against damage from free radicals. Copper is bound to the protein ceruloplasmin, which is a very important antioxidant in the blood. Ceruloplasmin prevents peroxidation (rancidity) of the polyunsaturated fats in cell membranes. An adequate intake of copper is also needed for healthy skin, hair, nails, and bones. It is involved in the production of collagen, a tough, fibrous, yet elastic, tissue found in bone, tendons, skin, and cartilage. Indeed, copper is a known folk remedy for arthritis; some people swear by their copper bracelets.

Symptoms of copper deficiency include anaemia, osteoporosis, and brittle, inflexible bones. There is a wide variation in dietary copper intake, and many women may be getting suboptimal amounts. This may not cause obvious symptoms, but it is a concern, given copper's vital role in maintaining bone and ligament integrity and in forming antioxidant reserves.

Good food sources of copper are animal liver, crustaceans, nuts, oysters, legumes, kidneys, fruits, and shellfish. You can also take copper in supplement form, as copper gluconate, copper sulphate, or copper amino acid chelate. The recommended dose is 1.5 to 3 milligrams daily. The ratio of copper to zinc taken in supplement form should be 1:10 – that is, if you take 30 milligrams of zinc, then the required dose of copper is 3 milligrams. However, if you have Wilson's disease – a rare hereditary syndrome characterized by an inability to metabolize copper properly – you should not take any copper supplements.

Magnesium

Magnesium is a mineral that has many important functions in the body. Among other things, it is involved in the production of enzymes and in the process by which cellular energy is released. Because it plays an important role in regulating muscular tone, it can serve as a natural muscle relaxant, making it useful for relieving such symptoms as muscle cramping and anxiety. Many menopausal women suffer from heart palpitations (an irregular or racing heartbeat) associated with hot flushes. This can be helped by increasing your intake of magnesium. Magnesium and calcium supplementation, in a ratio of two milligrams of calcium for each milligram of magnesium, can reduce bone loss after menopause. Magnesium is also essential for the health of the heart and the circulatory system (see page 154). An appropriate supplemental dose of magnesium is around 500 milligrams daily.

Manganese
Manganese is a vital mineral for health and is required for the metabolism of food and the production of sex hormones. Like copper, it is an antioxidant and is an element in superoxide dismutase, a potent antioxidant enzyme, and thus helps to reduce degenerative diseases associated with ageing. Manganese is also part of normal bone and cartilage structure, and can be helpful for sufferers of osteoarthritis. Some studies have found that women with osteoporosis have low levels of manganese compared with women whose bones are normal.

The National Research Council of America states that an adequate daily intake of manganese is 2 to 5 milligrams, and even up to 10 milligrams daily is safe. Good food sources of manganese are whole grains and nuts, wheat bran, organ meats, shellfish, and milk. Many fruits and vegetables contain moderate amounts, but this varies depending on the manganese content of the soil where they were grown. Manganese can be taken in supplement form as manganese gluconate or manganese amino acid chelate.

Selenium
Selenium is a trace mineral that is vital for good health. It is important in maintaining healthy immune function and tissue elasticity, including that of the skin and mucous membranes. It is also an important antioxidant that works synergistically with vitamin E to prevent free radical damage and support the health of the heart and circulatory system. (For information about the antioxidant actions of selenium, see Chapter 7.)

Silica

Silica is a form of the mineral silicon, which is the second most abundant element in the earth's outer layer. Silicon is used to make glass and computer chips, among other things, and in the last decade has been found to be an essential trace mineral for animals and for humans.

Silicon is found in human bone, fingernails, skin, and connective tissue, and adds mechanical integrity and hardness to their architectural matrix. Some researchers believe that silicon may offer some protection against atherosclerosis by strengthening connective tissue in the blood vessel walls.

The best food sources of silicon and silica are seafood, whole grains, and vegetables. If you consume a balanced diet, you probably get about 200 milligrams of silica daily. The herb horsetail is high in silica, and can be taken as a tea or in the form of an extract called vegetal silica. Silica can also be taken as part of a multimineral formula. Taking moderate amounts of supplemental silica has no known side-effects. The recommended dosage is 25 to 100 milligrams daily.

Zinc

Zinc is an essential mineral for the body, as more than 200 enzymes require zinc for their activity. It is also important for the proper functions of cell membranes. Zinc is vital for a healthy immune system and helps to keep hair, nails, and bones strong.

Good food sources of zinc include brewer's yeast, seafoods, whole grain products, wheat bran, lean meats, blackstrap molasses, liver, sesame and sunflower seeds, and oatmeal. Zinc can also be taken in supplement form as zinc amino acid chelate. Recommended supplemental doses for women are 15 to 30 milligrams daily. To avoid possible stomach upset, take zinc supplements with food, and do not exceed the recommended dosage, as the consumption of too much zinc may upset the balance of other necessary minerals in the body. It is best to take zinc on an intermittent basis, for example, three months on, three months off.

L-Glutamine

L-glutamine is an amino acid that crosses the blood–brain barrier and passes into the brain tissue, where it is converted into glutamic acid. The brain then converts glutamic acid into the neurotransmitter gamma-amino-butyric-acid (GABA). GABA is a neuroinhibitory transmitter that regulates many aspects of brain function. Around one-third of all the nerve cells in the brain send inhibitory, rather than accelerating, signals, and this is done via GABA.

Taking L-glutamine increases the production of GABA. This process can also be aided synergistically by taking 50 milligrams of vitamin B6 daily. Increased levels of GABA in the brain serve as a natural calming and memory-enhancing agent, and generally help one to think more clearly. L-glutamine is also useful for people who tend to use alcohol to help them cope with stress, as it reduces the craving for alcohol. The recommended dosage of L-glutamine is 500 milligrams, twice daily. It should be taken on an empty stomach, preferably with fruit juice.

Royal Jelly

Royal jelly is a natural food supplement that is rich in many essential vitamins, minerals, enzymes, hormones, and amino acids. It also contains antibiotic components. Royal jelly has energy-boosting properties, making it useful for symptoms of fatigue as well as for improving memory and overall mental and physical functioning. (For further information about royal jelly, see Chapter 9.)

Essential Fatty Acids

The health benefits of essential fatty acids are huge and diverse, and could be the subject of an entire book. Essential fatty acids (EFAs) are vital for the production and release of many hormones, including sex hormones and adrenal hormones. They are also an integral part of cell membranes, and they give these membranes proper flexibility and suppleness. They stop your cells from drying out and give them normal cohesiveness.

There are two basic types of EFAs, known as omega-3 and omega-6. These nutrients can help overcome dry, itchy skin, dry hair, hair loss, dry eyes, dry mouth, and can reduce vaginal dryness. They also help to reduce infections of the skin and mucous membranes such as cystitis, vaginitis, and mouth ulcers.

Many women use expensive creams and shampoos, to no avail; their skin and hair remain unhealthy. This is because they are lacking in EFAs. If you feed your skin and hair from within by using EFAs, you will be delighted with the difference – but give it time. It usually takes three to four months to see results.

Other benefits of EFAs include an improvement in the function of the nervous system, so I recommend them for women with a poor memory, insomnia, or mood disorders. Many women find that EFAs have the added benefit of reducing hot flushes, presumably because EFAs enhance and balance the production of sex hormones and prostaglandins. (For information about the role of EFAs in the production of prostaglandins, see Chapter 7.) EFAs exert an anti-inflammatory effect and can reduce the pain of arthritis and general muscular aches and pains.

Essential fatty acids must be obtained from foods like fish, fish oils, and unprocessed fresh vegetables, seeds, nuts, and botanical oils. To boost your intake of omega-6 EFAs, take 2,000 to 3,000 milligrams of evening primrose oil, 1,000 milligrams of lecithin, and 1,000 milligrams of spirulina daily. To increase your level of omega-3 EFAs, take 1,000 to 2,000 milligrams of fish oil capsules daily or increase your consumption of fish to four servings weekly. In addition, use one tablespoon of cold-pressed pure rape seed/canola, olive, or sunflower oil in your salad daily. Another tasty way to boost your levels of EFAs at breakfast time is to grind a mixture of linseeds, almonds, and sunflower seeds and sprinkle it on your cereal or rice (see page 147).

Herbs

There are many herbs that contain plant oestrogens or that act to stimulate the production of your natural hormones. These herbs can 'bridge the gap' between the time when your ovaries cease their oestrogen-producing function and when your adrenal glands start producing a different form of oestrogen, called oestrone. Oestrone is not as powerful as the oestrogen produced by the ovaries, which is called oestradiol; however, it is often enough to reduce unpleasant symptoms during this transition period.

Table 7 lists herbs that are suitable for use in menopause, with a brief overview of their actions, as well as information on how to use them. Herbs can be purchased from health food outlets or from a qualified herbalist.

The appropriate method of preparing a herbal remedy from fresh herbs depends on which part of the plant is used. The flowers and leaves of herbs may be prepared by making a tea. Bring water to a boil on top of the stove. While the water is boiling, place the herbs in a glass or ceramic (not metal) teapot that has a tight-fitting lid. Use 15 grams (approximately one tablespoon) of the dried herb to one cup of water. When the water boils, pour it over the herbs, cover and let the tea steep for ten to fifteen minutes. Then strain it and drink. You can sweeten the tea with a teaspoon of honey if needed.

If you are using the dried root, seeds, or woody parts of a plant, you will need to make what is called a decoction. Place 15 grams (about one tablespoon) of the dried herb in a glass or enamel (not metal) saucepan and add one cup of cold water. Let the herbs soak in the water for ten minutes, then cover the pot and bring it to a boil over high heat. Reduce the heat and let the mixture simmer for fifteen minutes. Then remove the pot from the heat and let the mixture steep for another ten minutes. Strain it and drink it warm.

Whether you are using a tea or a decoction, I recommend that a cupful be taken warm, not hot, three times a day.

TABLE 7 HERBS FOR MENOPAUSE

There are many medicinal herbs that can be helpful for the menopausal woman. This table lists those herbs that I have found to be most valuable, together with their actions and uses. These herbs should be available through a herbalist or at good health food stores.

HERB	PART USED	ACTIONS AND USES
Black cohosh (*Cimicifuga racemosa*)	Dried roots and rhizomes	This is a good oestrogenic herb that acts specifically on the uterus to reduce cramps and congestion. It is also good for relieving hot flushes. Black cohosh contains two anti-rheumatic agents and is excellent for relieving muscular pain and cramping. Take 250 mg in tablet or capsule form, two to four times daily. Or take 1/2 teaspoon of tincture, twice daily.
Chaste tree (*Vitex agnus-castus*)	Dried fruit	This herb is a hormone balancer that is used to alleviate depression at menopause. Take 300–600 mg in tablet or capsule form daily. Or take 1/2 teaspoon of tincture, twice daily.
Damiana (*Turnera diffusa*)	Dried leaves	Damiana is a great herb for menopause because it is a pituitary regulator and anti-depressant. It is also an aphrodisiac and is of benefit for sexual difficulties. It should not be taken too frequently, however, or it may irritate the lining of the urinary tract; I recommend taking 100–150 mg in tablet or capsule form, for two or three days out of the week. Or take 1/2 teaspoon of tincture, twice daily, for two or three days out of the week.
Dandelion (*Taraxacum officinale*)	Leaves, roots, and tops	Dandelion is a wonderful herb for the liver. If your hormones are out of balance, your liver is under extra stress, them dandelion root will be beneficial.

Herb	Part Used	Actions and Uses
Dandelion (cont.)		Take 1,000–3,000 mg in tablet or capsule form, or 2–3 cups of tea, daily. Or take 1–2 teaspoons of tincture, three times daily.
Dong quai (*Angelica inensis*)	Roots	This herb is high in natural plant oestrogens called phytosterols and helps to reduce the symptoms of oestrogen deficiency. Take 500 mg in tablet or capsule form, twice daily. Or take $1/2$ teaspoon of tincture, twice daily.
False unicorn root (*Chamaelirium luteum*)	Dried roots and rhizomes	This plant is an oestrogen regulator. It has a direct action on the uterus and ovaries and is considered to be a corrective herb for women. It is a specific for the herbal treatment of ovarian cysts. Take 500 mg in tablet or capsule form daily. Or take 1 teaspoon of tincture daily.
Ginkgo (*Ginkgo biloba*)	Leaves	This herb improves brain function, circulation, and oxygenation of all body cells. It is helpful for symptoms of fatigue, memory problems, and depression. Take 1,000 mg in tablet or capsule form daily. Or take 1 teaspoon of tincture, twice daily.
Ginseng (*Eleutherococcus senticosus, Panax quinquefolius*)	Roots	Ginseng strengthens the adrenal glands, enhances immune function, increases energy, and normalizes blood pressure. It is useful for symptoms of both mental and physical fatigue. Take 1,000–4,000 mg in tablet or capsule form daily. Ginseng is a safe energy-booster for most people. However, if you have very high blood pressure (over 180/100), you should avoid it. Siberian ginseng appears to be more effective than the American variety.
Liquorice (*Glycyrrhiza glabra*)	Dried roots and rhizomes	Liquorice is a powerful adrenal stimulant and is a wonderful oestrogenic herb. For this reason, it is a very useful herb

Herb	Part Used	Actions and Uses
Liquorice (cont.)		during menopause. Care must be taken, however, not to take liquorice too often, or it can deplete potassium and elevate blood pressure. If you have high blood pressure, use it with caution or avoid it entirely. On the other hand, if you suffer from low blood pressure, this herb will be useful in correcting the problem. Liquorice makes a pleasant-tasting tea. It can also be added in small amounts to other herbal teas to improve their flavour. For hot flushes, I recommend drinking 1–2 cups of liquorice tea or taking 500–1,000 mg in table or capsule form daily. Or take ½–1 teaspoon of tincture, twice daily.
Liferoot (*Senecio aureas*)	Dried plant	Liferoot is a uterine tonic that contains plant oestrogens. It helps to re-establish emotional and vascular stability and eliminate hot flushes. Take 500 mg daily in tablet or capsule form. Or take ½ teaspoon of tincture, twice daily.
Raspberry (*Rubus idaeus*)	Fresh or dried leaves and fruit	Raspberry is an astringent and nutritive oestrogenic herb. It has a direct action on the uterine muscles and helps to tone weakened muscles. It also assists in correcting prolapse of the uterus and/or vagina. Take 2,000 mg in tablet or capsule form or drink 2–3 glasses of raspberry tea daily. Or take ½–1 teaspoon of tincture, up to three times daily.
Red clover (*Trifolium pratense*)	Dried flower heads; fresh plant	Red clover contains a plant oestrogen called coumestrol and one of its medicinal actions is to stimulate the ovaries. It is a good alkalinizing herb described in herbals as an alterative, meaning that it restores healthy body functions. Red clover is a specific for the treatment of ovarian cysts. To relieve hot flushes, take 1,000–2,000 mg of red clover in tablet or capsule form or drink 3–4 cups of red clover tea daily. Or take ½–1½ teaspoons of tincture, up to three times daily.

Herb	Part Used	Actions and Uses
Sage (*Salvia officinalis*)	Fresh or dried leaves	This herb has many medicinal properties and is very useful during menopause for the treatment of hot flushes. Sage reduces excessive sweating and it contains plant oestrogens. You will find sage particularly useful in eliminating night sweats. Drink 3–4 cups of sage tea daily to relieve hot flushes, or take $^1/_2$–1 teaspoon of tincture, three times a day. Sprinkle finely chopped fresh sage in soups and on salads and vegetables.
St John's wort (*Hypericum perforatum*)	Fresh or dried flowering plant	This herb is a mild sedative that is specific for anxiety states. Take 500 mg in tablet or capsule form, or $^1/_4$–1 teaspoon of tincture, two or three times daily.
Sarsaparilla (*Smilas officinalis*)	Dried roots and rhizomes	Sarsaparilla is another alterative herb that stimulates the production of testosterone and therefore improves a flagging libido. Take 1,000–2,000 mg in tablet or capsule form or drink 2–3 glasses of sarsaparilla tea daily. Or take $^1/_4$–$^1/_2$ teaspoon of tincture, up to three times daily.
Saw palmetto (*Serenoa serrulata*)	Dried fruit	This herb is an astringent diuretic that is beneficial for the treatment of urinary incontinence, fluid retention, and prolapse of the pelvic organs. Dryness and lack of tone in the tissues of the bladder often lead to irritation and weakness. This is reduced by saw palmetto. Take 1,000–2,000 mg in tablet or capsule form daily. Or take $^1/_2$ teaspoon of tincture, twice daily.
Shepherd's purse (*Capsella bursapastoris*)	Dried flowering plant; fresh plant	Shepherd's purse is a pituitary regulator with androgenic properties. One of its primary attributes is its ability to normalize progesterone levels. If you are moving into menopause and have been experiencing excessive, irregular

HERB	PART USED	ACTIONS AND USES
Shepherd's purse (cont.)		bleeding or spotting, this herb will help to regulate and increase the length of your menstrual cycles until the natural cessation of menses. Take 500 mg in tablet or capsule form daily, or take ¼–½ teaspoon of tincture, up to twice daily.
True unicorn root (*Aletris farinosa*)	Dried roots and rhizomes	This oestrogenic herb stimulates and strengthens the female genital organs. It is a bitter herb that is also useful for indigestion and has a mild sedative action. Take 500–1,000 mg in tablet or capsule form daily. Or take ½ teaspoon of tincture, twice a day.
Wild yam (*Dioscarea villosa*)	Dried roots and rhizomes	Wild yam is a powerful oestrogenic herb used by women around the world. It has a good anti-inflammatory action and gives relief from menopausal arthritis. It also has progestogenic properties, and may help to reduce heavy menstrual bleeding. Take 1,000–4,000 mg of dried extract daily. Or take ½ teaspoon of tincture, twice a day.

If you do not have the time or inclination to prepare your own herbal teas, you may take herbs in dried form as tablets or capsules. Herbs are also available in the form of tinctures, which are liquid extracts, and dried extracts, which can be turned into tablets and capsules. Both tinctures and dried extracts are concentrated sources of herbs, so smaller amounts are required to achieve the same effect. In general, I recommend that herbs be taken in tea, tablet, or capsule form, rather than as tinctures, because tinctures contain varying concentrations of the active ingredient, they tend to be very strong-tasting, and they contain alcohol. Consult a qualified herbalist, or your local health food store for availability and for good, reputable brands of herbs. If you have difficulties obtaining information about natural therapies for menopause locally, write to me at the address at the back of this book.

STRATEGIES FOR HEALTHY BLOOD VESSELS

Naturopathic medicine is not only useful for treating the acute discomforts of the perimenopausal period, but also has a role to play in preventing or reducing some of the health problems that result from the lack of oestrogen over the long term. As discussed in Chapter 2, after menopause women are at significant risk of heart and blood vessel disease. Indeed, cardiovascular disease is the number one killer of women in Western societies, claiming twice as many lives every year as cancer. Although these diseases tend to attack women later then men, this should not stop women looking for ways to decrease their risk. Furthermore, the survival rate for women who suffer heart attacks is lower than that for men, regardless of age. Let us take a look at some of the nutritional strategies you can use to decrease your risk of cardiovascular disease. These good nutritional habits will also reduce your risk of cancer and obesity.

MINIMIZE FATS

Reducing the amount of fat in your diet will lower your risk of heart disease and cancer. Fats and oils are extremely high in calories, and if you eat excessive amounts of them, they slow down your metabolic rate, keeping you from losing weight and contributing to obesity.

Much of the fat in your diet can be eliminated simply by changing your habits and cooking techniques. One basic principle that will help to cut the amount of fat in your diet is to cut down on meat and dairy products and to increase the proportion of your diet that consists of grains. legumes, fruits, and vegetables. This will also take a load off your kidneys and help you retain calcium. Another way to lessen the amount of fat in your diet is to stop buying processed foods such as packaged biscuits, cakes, pastries, and fried foods, which are high in fat.

Avoid frying your foods (especially deep-frying!) and roasting or baking meats in their own fat. Grilling, boiling, steaming, and dry-baking are better. The one exception to this rule is stir-frying, which can be done with a minimum of added oil in a non-stick, non-aluminium pan. When you must use oil, use small amounts of cold-pressed vegetable oils such as pure rape seed/canola, olive, sunflower, or grapeseed, and cook your food slowly, at lower temperatures, to avoid having the oil become oxidized. Resist the temptation to add salt or use pre-packaged sauces; instead, flavour your foods with vegetable extracts, tomato purée, herbs, and spices.

When you select a prepared food product such as breakfast cereal, take the time to read the product information on the packaging. You may be surprised to find that some popular brands have very high levels of fat, salt, and sugar. Good low-fat alternatives to processed breakfast cereals are oatmeal and natural, unsweetened muesli, as well as barley and brown rice, which can be boiled and eaten as a hot cereal with the addition of a little low-fat milk.

You can also make an excellent mixture called LSA (for linseeds-sunflower seeds-almonds) that can be added to your breakfast cereal. Mix $1^1/_2$ cups linseeds, 1 cup sunflower seeds, and $^1/_2$ cup almonds together and grind them into a fine meal in a food processor or grinder. LSA is an excellent concentrated source of omega-6 essential fatty acids, fibre, natural plant oestrogens, protein, calcium, selenium, vitamin E, vitamin A, and the B vitamins. It must be kept fresh; store it in the refrigerator. Start making healthy choices and feel the benefit.

Saturated Fats

When reducing the amount of fat in your diet, it is important to know that all fat is *not* created equal. In particular, saturated fats are the most important ones to eliminate, as consuming excessive amounts of them can lead to obesity, clogged arteries, and an increased risk of cancer of the breast, ovaries, uterus, and bowel.

The easiest way to identify saturated fats is that they are solid at room temperature. Examples of saturated fats are those found in beef, pork, lamb, poultry, cheese, chocolate, butter, copha, suet and lard. Meat drippings, whole milk, cream, ice cream, and coconut and palm oils also contain saturated fats. I am not saying that you must avoid these foods completely, but you should keep your consumption of them to as low a level as possible. Make sure that you remove all the fat from meat and the skin from chicken, and use low-fat dairy products. You may safely eat two to three servings of red meat per week, provided you remove all the fat. Never fry red meat or chicken; bake or grill these meats or use them in casseroles and stews.

Eggs may be eaten in moderation, up to four per week. Eggs contain cholesterol, but they are also an excellent source of the sulphur-containing amino acids L-cysteine and L-methionine. L-cysteine contains a form of sulphur that inactivates free radicals and thus protects and preserves cells. It is also a precursor of glutathione, a major antioxidant in the body. L-methionine helps to eliminate fatty substances that can otherwise clog the blood vessels, and it is vital for efficient liver function, which helps to rid the body of toxins. The sulphur-containing amino acids found in eggs can thus be considered anti-ageing foods. Always boil or poach your eggs, rather than frying them; when fried, eggs produce oxycholesterol, or oxidizing cholesterol, a dangerous fat that generates free-radical production in the body.

Processed or delicatessen meats, such as processed luncheon meats, smoked or pressed ham, salami, pepperoni, etc., are not healthy to eat, as they are loaded with saturated fats. Moreover, because they are not fresh, their fats may become rancid. Rancid fats are highly oxidized and generate free radicals in the body that attack blood vessels and body cells. Also, these meat products contain nitrites, which have been linked to the development of cancer.

Cholesterol

Cholesterol is a pearly fatlike substance that is produced in your liver. It cannot dissolve in water or blood, so is transported in the bloodstream by specialized molecules called lipoproteins. Lipoproteins are not found in foods, but are manufactured by the liver, and they come in two basic types: high-density lipoproteins (HDL) and low-density lipoproteins (LDL). HDLs are scavengers that pick up free cholesterol in the blood and carry it back to the liver to be re-used or broken down. LDLs are larger than HDLs and are heavily laden with cholesterol, which they are supposed to transport to the body's cells, as needed.

Cholesterol is actually a necessary substance, and if you do not eat any foods that contain it, your body will make it. It becomes a problem, however, when there is more of it present than your body can cope with. Thus, if your diet contains a lot of cholesterol, it may end up being deposited on the walls of your arteries, leading to hardening and blockage of the arteries. To prevent this, it is necessary to have enough HDL circulating in your bloodstream to scavenge excess cholesterol and prevent it from causing harm. You can increase your levels of beneficial high-density lipoproteins by exercising regularly, reducing the amount of saturated fats in your diet, maintaining a healthy weight, and not smoking.

Your body can produce all the cholesterol you need without the need for added dietary cholesterol. If you consume very little dietary cholesterol, your need for high-density lipoproteins will also be low. Generally, it is ideal to have a cholesterol level of less than 5.5 mmol/Litre. In some people, elevated blood cholesterol may increase the risk of heart disease. Cholesterol is found mostly in foods of animal origin, such as meat, poultry, seafood, eggs, and dairy products. However, it is not only the amount of cholesterol but also the amount of saturated fats in the diet that affects a person's blood cholesterol level. This is because, when excessive amounts of saturated fats are eaten, the body responds by converting the fat into cholesterol. Foods high in saturated fats include all land animal products such as fatty meats, preserved meats, and whole-milk dairy foods; other sources are shellfish and coconut and palm oils.

Reducing dietary saturated fat is very important, but it is only one of the methods of reducing cholesterol levels. You must also increase your consumption of foods that help to lower cholesterol. These include oily fish (such as salmon, sardines, and tuna), vitamin-C-rich foods (citrus fruits, melons, cabbage, fresh green leafy vegetables, kiwi fruits, sweet and chili peppers, and strawberries), garlic, onions, and foods containing soluble fibre. Soluble fibre is fibre that dissolves easily in water and is found in the gums, pectin, and mucilages of plant fibre. Good sources of soluble fibre are legumes, cereals, whole grains, oat bran, fruits, and vegetables. Soluble fibre protects against gallstones, ulcerative colitis, high blood pressure, high blood cholesterol, and diabetes.

Unsaturated Fats

Unsaturated fats are fats that are liquid at room temperature. Examples are fish oils and olive, linseed, pure rape seed/canola, grape seed, peanut, corn, safflower, sesame, soyabean, and sunflower oils. These oils are combinations of monounsaturated and polyunsaturated oils. The best choices among these oils are olive, pure rape seed/canola, and linseed. This is because these oils contain large amounts of monounsaturated oils. Research has shown that these oils can be beneficial to the health of our arteries.[3] Mediterranean peoples have consumed these oils regularly for centuries, and have very low rates of heart disease.

Try to obtain cold-pressed vegetable and seed oils, as no fat or oil is healthy if it is subjected to heat processing or if food is fried in it. Both animal fats and vegetable oils, when they are heated to high temperatures, form chemicals that attack and destroy blood vessel walls.

If you use butter or margarine, do so only in moderation (if you are trying to lose weight, it is best to avoid these products altogether). Butter is a natural product, but it is high in cholesterol, saturated fat, and calories. Margarine is a synthetic product that is made by subjecting vegetable oils to a process called hydrogenation. This is what makes margarines solid or semi-solid at room temperature. However, hydrogenation also results in the creation of substances called cis- and trans-fatty acids. Cis- and trans-fatty acids are not useful nutritional substances and, if consumed regularly in large amounts, can have negative effects on your cardiovascular system. In addition, many brands of margarine contain other added chemicals to make them look and taste more like butter. Thus, while some people once thought that margarine was a healthy alternative to butter, it is now known that a small amount of butter is probably better for you than any amount of margarine. I recommend that you use a spread like tahini, avocado, or hummus instead of either margarine or butter.

Cut Down on Salt

Salt is a compound of two elements, sodium and chloride. Standard table salt consists of 40 per cent sodium and 60 per cent chloride. Our nutritional requirement for sodium is only 250 to 350 milligrams each day. One level teaspoon of salt contains 2,000 milligrams of sodium, so it is easy to see that many of us eat too much salt. Excess salt in the diet increases your risk of developing high blood pressure, cardiovascular disease, fluid retention, and osteoporosis.

Many menopausal women consume too much sodium. This is not surprising when you consider how much salt is added to processed and convenience foods, and that the salt and pepper shakers are standard additions to the dinner table.

There are several things you should do to reduce your sodium intake. Read labels on processed foods and avoid products that contain salt or sodium in any form. Watch for 'hidden' sodium, in the form of flavour enhancers and preservatives, such as monosodium glutamate (MSG), hydrolysed proteins, autolysed yeast, sodium caseinate, and calcium caseinate. Occasionally, MSG is included in salt shakers at fast food outlets or used to add a different flavour to French fries or chicken; it is a well-known addition to Chinese food. Other label terms that may indicate the presence of sodium in processed foods include malt flavouring, high-flavoured yeast, yeast extract, soyabean extract, textured soy

---

TABLE 8

PERCENTAGES OF FATTY ACIDS IN DIFFERENT OILS

Oils from vegetables, seeds, and nuts contain different mixtures of saturated, monounsaturated, and polyunsaturated fats. It is the chemical structure of a fatty acid that determines which class it belongs to. The consumption of saturated fats tends to raise cholesterol levels and has been linked to obesity, heart disease, and a number of different types of cancer. On the other hand, oils high in monounsaturated fatty acids, such as olive, canola, and avocado oil, are beneficial in that they can lower total cholesterol levels. Polyunsaturated fats are sources of essential fatty acids. This table illustrates the relative proportions of the types of fatty acids found in commonly used oils and vegetables.

OIL	PERCENTAGE OF SATURATED FATTY ACIDS	PERCENTAGE OF MONOUNSATURATED FATTY ACIDS	PERCENTAGE OF POLYUNSATURATED FATTY ACIDS
Avocado	10.0	70.0	10.0
Canola (rape seed)	6.0	60.0	34.0
Coconut	92.0	6.0	2.0
Linseed	6.0	24.0	70.0
Grape seed	11.1	17.3	71.6
Olive	10.0	82.0	8.0
Safflower	8.0	13.0	79.0
Sesame	13.0	46.0	41.0
Sunflower	8.0	26.0	66.0

protein, and even such harmless-sounding phrases as 'spices' or 'seasonings'. Artificial sweeteners can also contain high levels of sodium. Reducing your intake of processed and fast foods usually leads to a large reduction of dietary sodium levels.

Finally, stop adding salt to your cooking and put away the salt shaker! At first you will miss the salty taste. You may have strong cravings for salt for even the first few months, but they will pass.

Eventually, your taste buds will readjust and you will be able to taste the more subtle natural flavours of foods again.

NUTRITIONAL SUPPLEMENTS FOR A HEALTHY HEART

Vitamin A, vitamin C, vitamin E, beta-carotene, and choline, and the minerals zinc and selenium, are known as the antioxidant nutrients. They help to reduce damage to the blood vessels caused by free radicals. (For information about free radicals and antioxidants, see Chapter 7.) If possible, find a good-quality antioxidant tablet containing all of these nutrients. If not, you can take each component separately. I recommend that you take the following daily:

- 10,000 international units of vitamin A or 20 milligrams of beta-carotene.
- 4,000 milligrams of vitamin C with bioflavonoids.
- 100 to 500 international units of vitamin E.
- 30 milligrams of zinc chelate.
- 500 milligrams of choline.
- 50 micrograms of selenium.

Vitamin E is required for energy production and enables muscle cells to use oxygen (the fuel for energy) more efficiently. It is thus beneficial for athletic people and for those wanting to reduce symptoms of heart disease, such as angina and palpitations. Vitamin E reduces oxidant damage to LDL cholesterol and the blood vessel walls, thereby helping to keep your arteries unclogged and your blood flowing freely.

A study conducted at Boston's Brigham and Women's Hospital and the Harvard School of Public Health showed that daily supplementation with vitamin E in doses of 100 to 400 international units reduced the risk of heart attack by 25 to 50 per cent in both men and women.

Garlic is the most popular food herb in the world today. It contains compounds such as sulphur-containing amino acids, antioxidants, selenium, and allicin, which exert beneficial effects on the blood vessels and immune system. It acts as a natural body cleanser and antibiotic. Best of all, it reduces levels of LDL (the so-called 'bad cholesterol') and reduces the tendency to form blood clots. You may eat garlic fresh or cooked in food, or take odourless garlic capsules; 1,000 to 2,000 milligrams (one to two grams) daily is a suitable dose.

Magnesium is a mineral vital for heart muscle relaxation and improves metabolic function and energy production in the heart muscle and blood vessel walls.[4] Good dietary sources of magnesium are wheat germ, nuts, soyabeans, legumes, whole grains, all dark-green vegetables, and milk. You can also take magnesium tablets. Recommended doses are 400 to 800 milligrams daily.

The herbs ginkgo biloba and bilberry contain bioflavonoids that have a vitamin-C-like action and strengthen the capillaries (tiny blood vessels) in your cardiovascular system. They are available in tablet or capsule form at pharmacies and health food stores. You can take from 1,000 to 2,000 milligrams of ginkgo biloba and up to 1,000 milligrams of bilberry daily. The supplement coenzyme Q10 also plays an important role in energy production in the heart, brain, and body muscles. I recommend a daily dose of 100 to 500 milligrams.

FOODS FOR HEALTHY BONES

Osteoporosis, one of the most serious long-term consequences of oestrogen deficiency, is common among postmenopausal women, but it is not inevitable. Good nutrition, especially the consumption of adequate amounts of calcium and other minerals, has an important part to play in both preventing and in slowing the progression of this disease.

Generally speaking, for healthy bones, women require 800 to 1,000 milligrams of calcium daily. During pregnancy, lactation, and menopause, calcium needs increase to 1,000 to 1,500 milligrams daily.

Good food sources of calcium include dairy products, salmon, tuna, sardines (with the bones), green leafy vegetables, and tofu. Table 9 lists foods that are good sources of calcium. Check to see if your daily diet provides you with an adequate amount of calcium. If your diet falls short of this, or if you are not sure, take a good-quality calcium tablet to give you 1,000 milligrams of calcium daily.

One of the best food sources of calcium is milk. A cup of milk daily will give you a good start to meeting your calcium requirements. When it comes to cows' milk, I recommend a calcium-enriched milk which is low in fat and much higher in calcium than skimmed milk. If you are on a dairy-free diet, you may choose calcium-enriched soya milk instead. Some soya milks are calcium-enriched, while others are low in calcium, so read labels to be sure the product you choose is a good source of calcium.

There are a number of different supplemental sources of calcium. Bone meal, which comes from the ground bones of young animals, contains calcium from microcrystalline hydroxyapatite. Bone meal calcium is well absorbed, but it is possible for it to be contaminated with heavy metals such as lead. Calcium carbonate, which contains 40 per cent elemental calcium, is the most concentrated and cheapest form, but its absorption varies. Calcium lactate, calcium citrate, and calcium gluconate are less concentrated forms of calcium (containing around 15 per cent elemental calcium) but are better absorbed than the carbonate forms.

Some calcium supplements contain a mixture of different types of calcium to improve absorption. Many good calcium supplements contain vitamin D (cholecalciferol), which enhances the absorption of calcium from the intestines. Calcium is best absorbed when taken on an empty stomach, although if need be it can be taken with food.

It should not, however, be taken with high-fibre foods such as cereals, grains, and legumes, as this will reduce its absorption. It can be taken with dairy products, fruits, vegetables, or meats.

To test the absorbability of a calcium supplement, place it in vinegar at room temperature for half an hour and stir every few minutes. After this time, the supplement should be completely dissolved. If it isn't, then it won't dissolve in your stomach, either, and you should switch to another brand that passes the vinegar test.

Our bones contain magnesium and the trace minerals zinc, silica, boron, and manganese in addition to calcium, and studies suggest that adequate amounts of all these different minerals (see pages 133–8) are more effective than calcium alone at preventing bone loss. If your diet is not always perfect, I suggest that you take a trace mineral tablet that contains all of these minerals. Calcium and other mineral tablets are best taken last thing at night before going to bed.

In addition to making sure you obtain sufficient calcium and other minerals in your diet, avoid making dietary mistakes that can steal minerals from your bones. Keep your consumption of protein from animal sources (meat, fish, dairy products) to no more than 50 grams daily. This is the equivalent of the amount of protein found in a 180-gram serving of meat or fish plus one 250-ml glass of milk. Avoid foods that contain phosphorus or phosphate additives. These include many processed foods and fizzy soft drinks. If you

TABLE 9

FOOD SOURCES OF CALCIUM

Many different foods contain calcium, but some contain more than others. This table will give you an idea of which foods are the best sources of calcium. Use it to see whether your normal diet is providing you with the recommended 1,000 milligrams of calcium per day. If not, you should either include more calcium-rich foods in your diet or take supplemental calcium to make sure you get enough of the vital mineral.

FOOD	SERVING SIZE	MILLIGRAMS OF CALCIUM
Dairy Products		
Buttermilk	1 cup	285
Cheese		
Camembert	30 grams	110
Cheddar	30 grams	204
cottage	1 cup	135
cream	30 grams	23
feta	30 grams	140
mozzarella, part-skimmed	30 grams	207
Parmesan, grated	1 tablespoon	69
ricotta, part-skimmed	1/2 cup	335
Swiss	30 grams	219
Cows' milk		
low-fat (2 per cent)	1 cup	297
skimmed	1 cup	302
skimmed, powdered	1 tablespoon	130
whole	1 cup	291
Egg	1 large	25
Goats' milk	1 cup	350
Sour cream	1 tablespoon	16
Yoghurt, plain		
whole-milk	1 cup	275
non-fat-milk	1 cup	452

FOOD	SERVING SIZE	MILLIGRAMS OF CALCIUM
Fish		
Crabmeat, canned	90 grams	38
Flounder or sole, baked	90 grams	16
Haddock, grilled	90 grams	51
Oysters	1 cup	111
Salmon, pink, canned	90 grams	181
Sardines, canned, drained	90 grams	325
Shrimp or scallops, cooked	90 grams	39
Tuna, light, canned	90 grams	10
Nuts and Seeds		
Almonds, unsalted	30 grams (about 25 nuts)	70
Brazil nuts, unsalted	30 grams (7–8 nuts)	55
Pistachio nuts (unsalted)	30 grams (about 23 nuts)	40
Sesame seeds, ground (if seeds are not ground, calcium is unavailable)	30 grams	290
Sunflower seeds	30 grams	30
Walnuts, unsalted	30 grams (about 25 nuts)	30
Tahini	1 tablespoon	85
Legumes and Soya Products		
Baked beans	1/2 cup	60
Chickpeas	1/2 cup	75
Hummus	1 tablespoon	15
Kidney beans	1/2 cup	60
Lima beans	1/2 cup	40
Miso	1/2 cup	92
Peanuts, roasted	1/2 cup	54
Peanut butter	1 tablespoon	6
Soya milk	1 cup	10
Soya milk, calcium-enriched	1 cup	40
Soyabeans, cooked	1/2 cup	90
Tofu	1/2 cup	130
Fruits		
Apple	1 medium	10
Apricots, dried, uncooked	1 cup	100
Avocado	1 medium	26
Banana	1 medium	7

FOOD	SERVING SIZE	MILLIGRAMS OF CALCIUM
Blackberries, raw	1 cup	46
Blueberries, fresh, raw	1 cup	9
Cantaloupe	1/2 medium	29
Dates, whole, pitted	10 medium	27
Figs, dried	10 medium	269
Grapefruit	1/2 medium	14
Grapes, seedless	10 medium	5
Kiwi fruit	1 medium	20
Mango	1 medium	21
Orange	1 medium	30
Papaya	1 medium	72
Peach	1 medium	4
Pear	1 medium	20
Pineapple, fresh, cubed	1 cup	11
Prunes, uncooked	10 medium	43
Raspberries	1 cup	27
Rhubarb, cooked	1/2 cup	170
Strawberries	1 cup	27
Watermelon	10 cm wedge	30

Vegetables

FOOD	SERVING SIZE	MILLIGRAMS OF CALCIUM
Asparagus, fresh, cooked	1/2 cup	22
Beetroot	1/2 cup	15
Broccoli, fresh, cooked	1 medium spear	83
Brussels sprouts, fresh, cooked	1/2 cup	28
Cabbage, raw	1 cup	32
Cabbage, cooked, drained	1 cup	50
Carrots, fresh, raw	1 medium	19
Carrots, fresh, cooked	1/2 cup	24
Cauliflower, fresh, cooked	1/2 cup	17
Celery, fresh, raw	1 medium stalk	16
Chinese leaves/Pak choi, fresh, raw	1/2 cup	37
Courgettes, cooked	1/2 cup	12
Green beans, fresh, cooked	1/2 cup	29
Kale, fresh, cooked	1/2 cup	47
Mustard greens, cooked	1/2 cup	76
Onions		
raw	1 medium	30
cooked	1/2 cup	23
Peas, green, cooked	1/2 cup	19
Potato, baked, with skin	1 medium	20

Food	Serving size	Milligrams of calcium
Pumpkin, canned	1 cup	64
Sauerkraut	1/2 cup	36
Spinach	1/2 cup	50
raw, fresh	1/2 cup	27
cooked, drained	1/2 cup	130
Spring greens, cooked	1/2 cup	27
Squash, acorn or butternut, mashed	1/2 cup	52
Sweet potato, cooked	1 medium	32
Tomato	1 medium	6
Grains and Grain Products		
Barley, cooked	1 cup	17
Bulgur, cooked	1 cup	18
Bread, most types	1 slice	0
Breakfast cereal, most types	1 cup	5–30
Oatmeal, cooked	1 cup	19
Pasta, enriched, cooked	1 cup	10
Rice, brown, cooked	1 cup	20
Rice, white enriched, cooked	1 cup	23
Miscellaneous		
Basil, dried	1 teaspoon	32
Celery seed	1 teaspoon	38
Chocolate, milk, plain	30 grams	50
Cinnamon	1 teaspoon	28
Molasses		
blackstrap	1 tablespoon	137
light	1 tablespoon	33
Sugar, brown	1 tablespoon	12

consume beverages containing alcohol or caffeine, either eliminate these items from your diet or keep your consumption to a moderate or low level. (For further information on dietary risk factors, see Chapter 2.)

As a doctor who has treated menopausal women for twenty years, I have seen my attitudes change and evolve over time. In my early days, I believed that hormone replacement therapy was the crucial factor in helping women to cope with menopausal problems and improve their health. In later years, I came to see the vital importance of nutrition and natural medicine. By using specific nutritional supplements and reducing the amount of fat, salt, refined sugars, and chemical additives in your diet, you provide a much stronger foundation for long-lasting health, youthfulness, and vitality than HRT alone could ever provide. The re-energizing power of nutritional and herbal medicine will never cease to amaze you once you learn to use its tools.

CHAPTER SEVEN

SLOWING DOWN THE AGEING PROCESS

As a doctor, I find that a significant percentage of women are worried that the onset of menopause signals a sudden increase in their rate of ageing and that their looks will fade overnight. But this need not occur, if you learn how to reduce some of the things that tend to accelerate the ageing process.

The rate at which you age is determined by several factors. The ones you cannot control are your genetic inheritance and the age at which you pass through menopause. Factors over which you can exert control include exercise, diet, lifestyle, exposure to the sun's ultraviolet rays, and the health of your immune system.

EXERCISE

Exercise is vital for women in midlife. After menopause, the body's metabolic rate decreases, causing a tendency to gain weight easily.

Fifty per cent of postmenopausal women experience an increase in body weight of at least five kilograms, and in many cases much more. Ideally, you should do at least twenty to thirty minutes of aerobic exercise daily to stimulate your heart, blood circulation, and respiration. This can consist of doing aerobic exercise to music (at a gym or in your own home), swimming, doing aqua-aerobics, jogging, or working out on a stationary bicycle or stair-climbing machine.

If you have not done any aerobic exercise before, the process should be started gradually. Begin with five minutes a day and gradually increase the amount of exercise over a four-week period, until you reach thirty minutes daily. If you smoke or if you have any cardiovascular risk factors, such as obesity, high blood cholesterol levels, diabetes, high blood pressure, or a family history of heart disease, you should have a full fitness check-up, including a cardiac stress test, done by a medical doctor before you undertake any aerobic exercise. If you have arthritic joints or a back problem, aerobics, jogging, and strenuous weight-bearing exercise may aggravate pain and damage. In that case, modified yoga, tai chi, swimming, and walking would be excellent choices, as they stretch the joints gradually and keep the muscles in tone.

Many menopausal women find that aerobic exercise can be awkward because of stress incontinence. This means that when pressure in the abdomen is temporarily increased by exercise (or by straining, sneezing, coughing, etc.), urine is passed uncontrollably, soiling the underclothes. This often happens in menopause because a deficiency of oestrogen can cause the pelvic floor muscles to weaken and sag so that the bladder is not sufficiently supported. Exercises to strengthen the pelvic floor muscles can overcome stress incontinence in 40 to 50 per cent of cases (see Chapter 8).

EXPOSURE TO THE SUN

As far as ageing of the skin is concerned, there is nothing worse than the ultraviolet (UV) radiation from the sun. Of course, protection from this radiation should begin at a young age, but many women who are now menopausal were not taught about the harmful effects of the sun while they were growing up, so it is common to see sun-damaged skin in this age group.

There are two different types of ultraviolet rays, UVA and UVB rays. UVB rays are stronger in the middle of the day and in the summer, and are the major cause of sunburn and skin cancer. UVA rays are present regardless of the season and time of day, and although they do not usually cause sunburn, they do contribute to skin cancer and premature ageing, particularly with long-term exposure.

To protect yourself from the sun, whenever you are outdoors, use a sunscreen cream or lotion with a sun protection factor (SPF) of at least 15. If you are very fair skinned, red-haired, blonde, or blue-eyed, you will be safer choosing an SPF higher than 15. Whatever SPF you choose, look for products that specify *full spectrum protection*. This means that they screen out both UVA and UVB rays. Apply the sunscreen to all exposed areas of skin every two hours—more often if you are swimming or perspiring a lot. Avoid spending time outdoors between 10 a.m. and 3 p.m., when UVB rays are strongest. In addition to sunscreen, wear a broad-brimmed hat and protective clothing, making sure to protect your neck and face, as these areas really show your age. Use good-quality sunglasses that specify broad-spectrum UV protection to filter out the ultraviolet rays.

THE ANTI-AGEING DIET

A woman in midlife need not be fanatical about diet, as obsessions can cause an early death through stress or boredom. However, there are four basic principles that should be followed for profound and far-reaching benefits to your physical and mental well-being. These principles are:

1 Learn to love *raw* vegetables and fruits. Ideally, around 50 per cent of your diet should consist of raw foods. Raw foods are living foods, and by virtue of this they stimulate the metabolism and aid in the elimination of toxic waste materials from the body. Raw foods contain beneficial molecules such as antioxidants and indoles, which have anti-cancer properties and are excellent for overcoming obesity, arthritis, and high blood pressure.

Ideally, a woman in midlife should buy herself a juice-extracting machine with which to make raw vegetable and fruit juices on a daily basis. Juices not only supply essential minerals and vitamins, but also contain easily assimilated organic compounds such as vegetable amino acids, which improve digestion, have natural antibiotic properties, and promote healthy intestinal flora. This reduces bad breath. Raw fruit and vegetable juices are distinct and incomparable in their rejuvenating and regenerating effect on the human organism. No other source supplies as much vitamin C as fresh fruits and vegetables do, and this vitamin is entirely destroyed when the juices are subjected to heat.

Generally, 500 ml of juice daily is the smallest amount that will yield worthwhile results. If you can manage more, so much the butter; 1 litre may be needed to stimulate a quicker process of detoxification and rejuvenation.

Recommended juices include:

- A combination of two or more of the following: apple, grapefruit, orange, strawberry, pear, pineapple, and peach.
- A combination of two or more of the following: carrot, celery, tomato, parsley, cucumber, cabbage, spinach, beet, radish, dandelion, lettuce, turnip green, and watercress.

For a healthy cocktail, add a dash of lemon, strawberry, and honey to either of the above recipes.

2 Avoid chemically processed and frozen foods and buy foods in their natural state. Fresh foods in their natural state contain fewer bacteria than processed frozen foods and thus promote healthy intestinal flora and good digestion, and reduce bad breath. Natural foods also contain more fibre, vitamins, and minerals; fewer calories; and less fat. Choose unprocessed grains, cereals, seeds, nuts, legumes, and whole-grain bread instead of products made with white flour, sugar, sweeteners, colourings, salt, commercial sauces, and hydrogenated oils. In addition to lacking any nutritional value, many artificial food additives are suspected of causing health problems ranging from allergies to headaches to cancer. Refined sugar and its various relatives (such as brown sugar and corn syrup) add little to the diet except calories. Furthermore, they cause your blood sugar level to rise very rapidly, and then to fall again just as rapidly. Such wild fluctuations in blood sugar can lead to lethargy and headaches, as

well as aggravating many unpleasant menopausal symptoms.

3 Reduce your intake of fats. This means reducing not just cholesterol, but all fats, especially saturated fats. Avoid fatty meats such as lamb, pork, ham, bacon, chicken with the skin, and processed meats, as well as fried foods, coconut, processed margarines, and whole-milk dairy products. You should especially avoid fats that have turned rancid. Oils that have been subjected to very high temperatures (repeated deep-frying, for example) and oils that are not fresh are likely to become rancid. Rancidity leads to the production of free radicals, which increase inflammation and promote the development of cancer (see below). Substitute monounsaturated and polyunsaturated fats for saturated fats by eating foods such as grilled fish, canned fish, tahini, hummus, seeds, grains, legumes, almonds, vegetables, and cold-pressed vegetable and seed oils.

4 Drink eight to twelve glasses of water daily. The best type of water is pure bottled water or water that has passed through a reverse osmosis filter system attached to your kitchen tap. If you live in an area that is generally free of air pollution, pure rainwater is an option as well. Water dilutes the blood, thereby reducing cholesterol and acidity and improving sluggish circulation. It helps to flush toxins from all of the body's tissues, reducing your body's exposure to these substances. It also improves kidney function and lowers blood pressure.

ANTIOXIDANTS

To understand the process of ageing, it is essential that you know about *free radicals*. These sound like political terrorists, and indeed they are dangerous, unstable electronic particles and terrorize our cells. They rush around the body damaging cell walls, genetic material, blood vessel walls, joints, and intracellular components.

When free radicals are produced in your skin, they damage the collagen, a protein that is an essential component of skin tissue and is responsible for the skin's elasticity. Free-radical damage causes cross-linkage and degeneration of collagen fibres, resulting in wrinkling, thinning, and ageing of the skin. These evil free radicals cause an atomic-bomb-type chain reaction in our precious cells that keeps on generating more and more free radicals. Obviously, we all hate free radicals, as they damage our cells, leading to more rapid ageing. All of us would like to reduce the production of free radicals in our bodies.

To some degree, free radicals are inevitable. They are formed when we are exposed to polluted air, cigarette smoke, rancid dietary fats, some highly processed chemical foods, fluorescent lights, video display units, viruses, and alcohol, among other things. But there is still a great deal we can do to protect our cells against their destructive effects.

Antioxidants are substances that scavenge and neutralize free radicals. They act as a defense system for our cells. Because they prevent and reduce cell damage, they help to prevent degenerative diseases and to slow down the ageing process. There are a number of different kinds of substances that act as antioxidants, including vitamins, minerals, enzymes, and amino acids. Some of the most potent are vitamin A, C, and E, and choline; the amino acids methionine and cysteine; and the mineral selenium. Many of these, you will notice, are the same nutrients that are recommended for easing the acute symptoms of menopause (see Chapter 6), so they really offer dual benefits.

Vitamin E

One of the best ways to protect our tender tissues from free-radical damage is to take vitamin E supplements. Vitamin E was the first recognized antioxidant. It has been known for many years for its anti-ageing effects, since long before scientists knew of the existence or understood the significance of free radicals.

One word of caution, however: only natural forms of vitamin E are useful. Unfortunately, thousands of women erroneously take synthetic forms of vitamin E, which are of negligible use. The natural forms of vitamin E are called dextro-tocopherols (or d-tocopherols). These d-tocopherols are a mixture of alpha, beta, gamma, delta, eta, epsilon, and zeta tocopherols (different variants of natural vitamin E that have slightly different chemical configurations), and they all play valuable roles in scavenging and neutralizing free radicals. D-alpha-tocopherol is the most common natural form of vitamin E sold in supplement form. Synthetic vitamin E is denoted by dl-alpha-tocopherol. The natural forms of vitamin E are 30 per cent more active (that is, effective) as antioxidants. Doses of 500 to 1,000 international units of vitamin E a day can help to slow down the ageing process. Vitamin E is also present in fresh wheat germ, nuts, and eggs, and in cold-pressed vegetable oils such as soyabean, olive, sunflower, sesame, and safflower oil.

According to Dr Jeffrey Blumberg, a cancer specialist at Tufts University in Boston, the incidence of cancer could be cut in half if people increased their consumption of antioxidants by making dietary changes and taking nutritional supplements. Vitamin E can inhibit the development of cancer of the skin, breast, and colon. Dr Blumberg has found compelling evidence that you can add years to a healthy life by taking sufficient antioxidants. He recommends taking supplements of vitamins A, C, and E, or eating between five and nine servings of fresh vegetables each day.

BETA-CAROTENE AND VITAMIN A

Another free-radical fighter is the nutritional substance called beta-carotene, which is found in high concentration in certain vegetables, such as carrots, beet greens, sweet potatoes, and pumpkin. That is one of the reasons why raw vegetable juices are so wonderfully good for age-conscious folks. If you consume too much beta-carotene, your skin may turn a slightly yellow or bronze colour, as carotene is a yellow pigment. This is harmless and is not equivalent to vitamin A overdosage. If it happens, simply reduce your intake of beta-carotene until the bronze colour fades.

It is possible to take beta-carotene in supplement form. A dose of 5,000 international units (six milligrams) can safely be taken one to three times daily. Beta-carotene is converted in the liver into vitamin A, which is beneficial because vitamin A is itself a powerful free-radical scavenger and so a useful anti-ageing substance. It is especially important for the strength and metabolism of the skin and mucous membranes, which are particularly vulnerable to drying and infection in menopausal women. As an alternative to beta-carotene, daily doses of 5,000 to 10,000 international units of vitamin A are generally helpful and safe. However, if you suffer from any medical disorders, check with your doctor first before taking vitamin A.

Vitamin C

The miraculous anti-ageing and rejuvenating properties of vitamin C are to the water-soluble parts of your body (such as intracellular fluid and serum) what vitamin E is to the fatty parts (such as cell membranes). Vitamin C is a powerful antioxidant and free-radical scavenger and is extremely important in maintaining the integrity of the collagen in your skin and bones and thus the elasticity of these tissues. Vitamin C reduces the rate of ageing of the skin and bones.

The best sources of vitamin C are fresh fruits and vegetables, but as a nutritional 'insurance policy', I recommend that all women take a daily supplement of 1,000 to 2,000 milligrams of vitamin C in the form of calcium ascorbate, which is easily dissolved in raw fruit and vegetable juices. Calcium ascorbate is **non-acidic and so is better for people who find the ascorbic acid form of vitamin C too acidic, and it is the best type of vitamin C** supplement for menopausal women because it also provides some calcium. Some people become hypersensitive or allergic to vitamin C supplements, even esterified vitamin C ('Ester-C'), which is normally well tolerated. If this happens to you, make sure you eat plenty of foods high in vitamin C, such as fresh raw fruits and vegetables.

According to Dr Judie Walton, a gerontologist at the Ageing Research Institute at Concord Hospital in Sydney, Australia, vitamins A and C are known to prolong life in experimental animals, and she expects that the same will be shown to be true for humans. Dr Walton says that this is logical as, if the antioxidant vitamins protect specialized cells (such as those of the brain, heart, liver, lungs, blood and immune system), these cells will not need to be replenished so often from our cell banks. The cell banks are stores of undifferentiated (primitive) cells found in the bone marrow, spleen, liver and blood. These primitive cells are used to replace dead cells throughout the body. If body cells do not need to be replenished as often, the cell banks should thus last longer and the individual's life span should increase accordingly.

SELENIUM

Selenium is an essential trace mineral that is essential for optimal health. It is also an important antioxidant. The body uses selenium to produce an intracellular antioxidant enzyme called glutathione peroxidase. This enzyme reduces oxidant damage to cell membranes, to the nucleic acids DNA and RNA, and to cell proteins, and thus is an ally in the fight against ageing. Adequate selenium is vital for this enzyme to function effectively. Selenium can provide useful protection against cancers, especially breast cancer, and a large range of degenerative diseases.

The best food sources of selenium are brewer's yeast, garlic, mushrooms, celery, onions, radishes, fish, grains, broccoli, cabbage, cucumbers, and organ meats, although the potency of these foods as sources of selenium may vary tremendously, depending on soil conditions in the places where they were produced. Selenium can be taken in supplement form, as inorganic sodium selenite, or in organic form in the foods mentioned above or in a special brewer's yeast enriched with selenium. Organic forms are probably preferable. Daily doses range from 50 to 200 micrograms of selenium.

ESSENTIAL FATTY ACIDS

Essential fatty acids (EFAs) are components of unsaturated fats that are necessary for health and vitality. They are termed essential for two reasons:

1   Our bodies are unable to manufacture them.
2   Our cells cannot function normally without them.

If a patient of mine asks me what the most important supplement is for health and beauty, I respond, 'Essential fatty acids'. This is because the membranes that surround and protect each cell in the body are made of essential fatty acids (see Figure 16). The physical integrity and energy production of our cells depends upon adequate amounts of essential fatty acids in the diet.

Cytoplasm

Cell membrane made of essential fatty acids

Cell nucleus

Figure 16 **A body cell**

If our cell membranes break down or weaken, they may no longer be able to prevent dangerous particles (toxic chemicals, infectious organisms, viruses, and free radicals, among others) from passing through them. If such dangerous particles manage to pass through a weakened cell membrane, they enter the 'inner sanctum' of the cell, where they may inflict severe damage. Such damage may be irreparable and result in physical, chemical, and electrical impairment of the cell. If cellular damage is widespread, it can result in chronic inflammation and degeneration, as well as increasing the rate of ageing of the cells. If a cell's nucleus, which contains the genetic control centre of the cell, is severely damaged, the cell may be transformed into a cancer cell. So you can understand why it is vital to have strong, healthy membranes around your cells to protect them. This is one of the most important strategies for slowing down the ageing process and enabling us to look, feel, and act younger longer.

Essential fatty acids are the most important nutrients for building and maintaining strong and efficient cell membranes. The antioxidants – vitamins A, C, and E, beta-carotene, and selenium – also help our cell membranes to keep out nasty invaders like free radicals and viruses. To use an analogy, one might think of a body cell as a castle. The cell membrane is the moat and brick wall around the castle; antioxidants are the defending army, shooting arrows from the parapets to weaken and repel the castle's invaders.

There are two types, or families, of beneficial EFAs: omega-6 and omega-3. Omega-6 EFAs are linoleic and gamma-linolenic acids. Omega-3 EFAs are alpha-linolenic and eicosapentaenoic acids.

EFAs not only strengthen cell membranes, but they also help to optimize the balance between vitally important hormone-like chemicals called prostaglandins. There are three families of prostaglandins: prostaglandin 1, prostaglandin 2, and prostaglandin 3. Let's call them PG_1, PG_2, and PG_3.

The PG_1 and PG_3 families are beneficial to the body because they reduce inflammation and regulate the function of many hormonal glands and also the brain's chemistry. As outlined in Table 10, omega-6 EFAs are used by the cells to produce PG_1, and omega-3 EFAs are used to produce PG3. The production of beneficial PG1 and PG3 is desirable and promotes a healthy immune system. In particular, PG1 acts as a powerful messenger in the body and increases the production and release of many different hormones, including thyroid hormone, cortisone, growth hormone, and sex hormones, as well as of neurotransmitters (brain chemicals that transmit messages from one nerve cell to another). Thus, omega-6 EFAs, by increasing PG1, keep your hormonal glands and brain cells 'switched on'. Because of this, a woman with mental fatigue, emotional imbalances, chronic fatigue syndrome, or adrenal gland exhaustion should take omega-6 EFAs to boost her PG1 levels.

Where can you obtain EFAs? They can be found in certain foods (such as fish, grains, beans, and seed oils) as well as in nutritional supplements. The best way of increasing your intake of EFAs is to take daily supplements of evening primrose oil (2,000 to 4,000 milligrams), linseed meal (two tablespoons of ground seeds), blackcurrant seed oil (1,000 milligrams), and/or fish oil (1,000 milligrams). Also, include fresh and canned fish, seeds, vegetables, and cold-pressed seed oils in your diet regularly. EFAs are vulnerable to damage from high temperatures, light, air, or hydrogenation, which makes them unusable by the body. In particular, the body cannot transform damaged EFAs into prostaglandins. That is why the best oils are those that are extracted from their source using a cold-pressed or expeller-pressed process, and that are not refined with chemicals, bleaches, solvents, or deodorants. Seeds or olives that are passed through a screw press, for example, release their oils without having to be subjected to high temperatures. Oils that are not filtered excessively retain more source nutrients.

Hydrogenated margarines, fried foods, and commercially processed oils all contain damaged fats. Many commercial cookies, pastries, cakes, crackers, and cereals also contain unhealthy fats, such as highly saturated palm and coconut oils, hydrogenated vegetable shortening, and margarine. Avoid these unhealthy fats, and try to use only unrefined cold-pressed monounsaturated or polyunsaturated oils.

Increasing your intake of EFAs can help you in many ways:

- Improving the appearance and health of your skin, hair, and nails.
- Increasing your mental and physical energy.
- Boosting your immune system.
- Reducing inflammation and aches and pains.
- Improving your circulation and reducing your chance of developing cardiovascular disease (or, if you already suffer from cardiovascular disease, reducing its severity).
- Reducing cellular damage, thereby slowing the rate of ageing and reducing your risk of developing cancer.
- Reducing breast pain and tenderness.
- Improving gynaecological health by reducing menstrual cramps, ovarian cysts, and pelvic inflammation.

As you age, your body becomes less efficient at manufacturing PG_1 and PG_3, and this is partly why you may slow down and suffer increasing aches and pains with advancing years. Also, as you age – and especially if your diet is high in saturated fats – you produce increasing amounts of the undesirable PG_2 family of prostaglandins. PG_2 promotes the body's inflammatory response, so its action tends to increase inflammation and pain. You can reduce the amounts of undesirable PG_2 in your body by reducing your total fat (especially saturated fat) intake, maintaining normal body weight, not overeating, and ensuring adequate intake of omega-3 and omega-6 EFAs, the B vitamins, zinc, and vitamins C and E. Many menopausal and postmenopausal women complain of a variety of painful syndromes, such as headaches, arthritis, rheumatism, and backaches. This is largely due to an imbalance in prostaglandins – too much PG_2 and not enough PG_1 and PG_3. In such cases, doctors may prescribe anti-inflammatory drugs known

TABLE 10

SOURCES AND FUNCTIONS OF FATTY ACIDS

This table provides an overview of selected fatty acids, together with the types of prostaglandins they are used to produce, the effects of these prostaglandins on the body, and food sources of the fatty acids. The correct balance of fatty acids – specifically, more omega-3 and omega-6 essential fatty acids and less arachidonic acid – is needed to create the optimal balance of prostaglandins in the body.

PROSTAGLANDIN FAMILY PRODUCED FROM THESE FATTY ACIDS	ACTIONS OF THESE PROSTAGLANDINS IN THE BODY	FOOD SOURCES OF THESE FATTY ACIDS
Linoleic Acid and Gamma-Linolenic Acid (Omega-6 Essential Fatty Acids)		
PG_1 (desirable)	Reduce pain and inflammation; improve skin; increase energy and vitality.	Breast milk; sesame, safflower, cotton, and sunflower seeds and oil (cold pressed); corn and corn oil; soya beans; raw nuts; legumes; leafy greens; blackcurrant seeds; and their oil; evening primrose oil; borage oil; gooseberry oil; spirulina; lecithin.
Alpha-Linolenic Acid and Eicosapentaenoic Acid (EPA) (Omega-3 Essential Fatty Acids)		
PG_3 (desirable)	Reduce pain and inflammation; help circulation.	Fresh fish from cold, deep oceans (such as mackerel, tuna, herring, flounder, sardines, salmon); rainbow trout; bass. Fish must not be fried. Also, linseed oil; blackcurrant and pumpkin seeds and their oil; cod liver oil; shrimp; oysters; leafy greens; canola oil; soyabeans; walnuts; wheat germ; wheat sprouts; fresh sea vegetables; fish oil capsules.

PROSTAGLANDIN FAMILY PRODUCED FROM THESE FATTY ACIDS	ACTIONS OF THESE PROSTAGLANDINS IN THE BODY	FOOD SOURCES OF THESE FATTY ACIDS
Arachidonic Acid (AA) **(Omega-6 Nonessential Fatty Acid)**		
PG2 (undesirable)	Excess amount may increase pain and inflammation and can result in excessively sticky blood platelets and poor circulation.	Animal meats; whole-milk dairy products; preserved meats; fried food; processed and takeaway foods; coconut and palm oils.

as antiprostaglandins, such as naproxen (Naprosyn) and diclofenac sodium (Voltarol), to suppress the body's production of PG2. These drugs work quickly and effectively to relieve pain and inflammation, but if taken for many months, they may cause unpleasant side-effects.

If my patients complain of pain and inflammation in their muscles, bones, and joints, I prefer to teach them how to reduce these problems with nutritional medicine, rather than having them rely on anti-inflammatory drugs alone. And this is not hard to do. Simply:

● Reduce the amount of saturated fats in your diet.
● Increase the amount of omega-3 and omega-6 essential fatty acids in your diet (see Table 10).
● Take antioxidant supplements daily.
● Take vitamin B complex and zinc supplements at least twice weekly.
● Drink one to two litres of water and at least 500 ml of raw vegetable juices daily.

The essential fatty acid story sounds too good to be true. However, I have recommended EFAs to thousands of women in poor health, and I can assure you that it is worth while to increase the amount of EFAs in your diet. As you grow older, you need to 'oil' – but not to 'grease' – to slow down the ageing process.

If you would like to know more about research into EFAs, you can write to Stephen Wright, MD, at the Royal Free Hospital & School of Medicine, Pond St., London NW3 2QG. Or refer to *Heal Cancer* by Ruth Cilento, MD, and/or *Making Fats and Oils Work for You* by Lewis Harrison.[1]

BOOSTING YOUR IMMUNE SYSTEM

Your immune system is the surveillance and defence system that protects your cells against infections, toxins, free radicals, and damage from such factors as radiation exposure (including sun exposure), poor diet, stress, cancer, and exposure to chemicals. The immune system is very complex and involves the lymphatic system, liver, spleen, bone marrow, and thymus gland. The thymus gland, situated in the lower part of the neck and behind the breastbone, or sternum, is the master gland of the immune system and orchestrates the activities of the other parts.

Unfortunately, the valuable thymus gland shrinks with age, leading to a general reduction in the efficiency of the immune system. As your ageing immune system weakens, you become more susceptible to degeneration and inflammation of the cells, infections, cancer, and even more rapid ageing. All of these things combined may eventually shorten your lifespan.

Thus you can comprehend the huge importance of a healthy immune system in the quest for youthfulness and a longer lifespan. The immune system acts to reduce damage and ageing of the most vulnerable parts of our cells, such as the nuclei and intracellular metabolic structures.

There are many simple, commonsense measures you can take to promote the health of your immune system:

● Avoid exposure to tobacco smoke, both from smoking and from secondhand smoke.

- Avoid exposure to toxic chemicals such as pesticides and solvents.
- Avoid engaging in high-risk behaviour such as intravenous drug use, unprotected sexual activity, and poor hygiene, all of which increase the risk of unnecessary infection.
- Avoid unnecessary surgery. Always get a second opinion before agreeing to any non-emergency surgical procedure.
- As much as possible, avoid stress. Steer clear of vexatious people and situations! Learn stress management techniques to help you cope with problems that are not avoidable.
- Keep the amount of fat in your diet to a minimum.
- If you drink alcoholic beverages, keep your consumption to a moderate level (no more than four to five drinks weekly).
- Avoid exposure to radiation, including excessive sun exposure and unnecessary X-ray or bone scan procedures. When using a computer, try to keep a distance of 70–90 centimetres away from the screen, and 120 centimetres from the back and sides of the unit; when watching television, sit at least 120 centimetres from the set. If you use a microwave oven, check it periodically to make sure the door seals tightly, and step back at least two metres from it when it is on. Avoid over-using microwave ovens as their long-term risks are unknown.
- Avoid excessive use of xenobiotic (non-organic) drugs, especially painkillers, sedatives, and anti-inflammatory drugs.
- Avoid consuming foods that contain chemical preservatives, colourings, and flavourings, such as artificial sweeteners.
- Investigate your local environment. If possible, try not to make your home in an area that is highly polluted or located near such potential hazards as power generators or coal mines.
- Maintain a body weight appropriate for your height and build.
- Eat plenty of raw fruits and vegetables, whole grains, and legumes.
- Take antioxidant supplements (see page 166).
- Make sure to get an adequate amount of sleep, at least six or eight hours a night for most people.

- Get regular exercise (see page 162).
- Make time for relaxation and pleasurable activities on a regular basis.
- Drink plenty of water and fresh juices, a total of two litres a day.
- Be yourself. Don't be afraid to assert your needs and talk about your feelings. Repressed emotions can increase the stress on your immune system.

If you take these simple measures to boost your immune system, you are likely to be rewarded with a healthier, happier life, and quite possibly a longer one.

ANTI-AGEING HORMONES

The body produces a number of natural hormones, such as growth hormone, thyroid hormone, and sex hormones, that help to keep us younger. They do this by maintaining muscular and skeletal mass, cardiovascular function, metabolism, and general function.

GROWTH HORMONE

One powerful hormone involved in the ageing process is growth hormone, which is produced by the pituitary gland. In the normal course of life, growth hormone production starts to decrease at the age of about twenty, and it continues to decline thereafter, reaching very low levels in some people by the age of sixty. This is usually accompanied by a reduction in muscle mass, metabolic rate, muscle strength, and exercise performance, and an increase in blood cholesterol level. Normal ageing is growth-hormone-related. A deficiency of growth hormone causes fatigue; an increase in body fat, especially around the stomach; a slight reduction in muscle mass; cold hands and feet; a tendency to feel cold; and sometimes sexual dysfunction. Growth hormone deficiency effects men and women in equal numbers.

There is no question that people with abnormally low levels of growth hormone should receive treatment. Recently, American scientists obtained excellent results from giving injections of growth hormone to a group of healthy but growth-hormone-deficient men. In a study reported by Drs Daniel Rudman, Axel Feller, and their co-workers in *The New England Journal of Medicine*, twenty-one healthy men from sixty-one to eight-one years of age with low levels of growth hormone were studied.[2] They were representative of the approximately one-third of all men in that age category who have subnormal levels of growth hormone. Twelve of the men were given injections of growth hormone for six months, and nine received no treatment.

The injections of growth hormone produced significant increases in lean body mass, spinal bone density, and skin thickness, with decreases in adipose (fat) tissue mass. In the nine men not on any growth hormone treatment, there were no significant changes. Six months of treatment with human growth hormone had an effect on lean body mass and adipose tissue mass that was equivalent in magnitude to the changes that normally take place in the course of ten to twenty years of ageing.

The conclusion of the study was that diminished secretion of growth hormone is responsible in part for the decrease of lean body mass, the expansion of adipose tissue mass, and the thinning of the skin that occur in old age. This concept is supported by beneficial results of growth hormone treatment in growth-hormone-deficient adults. We know that injections of growth hormone can increase lean body tissue, muscle mass, and exercise performance, while reducing body fat and blood cholesterol. Still, questions about costs, benefits, safety, and side-effects must be critically examined before growth hormone can be considered for general use in ageing populations.[3]

You will be happy to know, however, that regular exercise **seems to promote the production of growth hormone by the pituitary gland. Simply by exercising regularly, you can slow down** the ageing process by increasing your own supply of precious growth hormone in a natural way.

THE THYMUS GLAND

Exciting new research in Europe and the United States shows that injections of extracts from the thymus gland may increase the resistance of the immune system to all disease in animals. When these injections have been used in human beings, they have often produced a feeling of rejuvenation in the recipients. Further research could very well reveal that taking extracts of thymus will slow down the ageing of the immune system.

THE THYROID GLAND

It is not uncommon for the thyroid gland to become slightly underactive at the time of menopause. Indeed, women are far more prone to thyroid disease than men are. The thyroid gland controls the metabolic rate, and if it becomes underactive, the metabolic rate will decline, causing easy weight gain, difficulty in losing weight, dryness and thickening of the skin, dryness and thinning of the hair, constipation, sensitivity to cold, and mental slowness.

The functioning of the thyroid gland can be checked by a simple blood test. If your thyroid is found to be underactive, you will most likely be prescribed thyroid hormone, which will re-establish your metabolic rate and cause a return to normal body weight and mental activity. If your metabolism is a little sluggish and you seem to have trouble burning up the calories, yet your blood test shows that your thyroid gland is functioning within normal limits, you may be able to stimulate your metabolism by taking spirulina (a nutritional supplement) and macrobiotic dried seaweed preparations. These contain the essential mineral iodine along with other minerals that generally stimulate the metabolism.

The subject of ageing is a fascinating one. Although we have made huge advances in understanding the factors that accelerate ageing, we still cannot prevent it; we can merely slow it down. Still, this is a formidable achievement in itself. I hope that you will utilize the suggestions in this chapter about diet, exercise, nutritional supplements, and boosting your immune system to add both years to your life and life to your years. Life's main problem is, after all, its brevity. Even if we manage to avoid such hazards as nuclear war, poisonous spiders, and dull people, our biblical lot still totals only around 620,000 hours. This does not even give us the satisfaction of being 'hour millionaires'. Every hour is precious, and anything that we can do to add a few extra is well worth our effort.

Chapter eight

Sex and Menopause

My patient Julie had had a hysterectomy for fibroids at the age of forty-seven. Two years later she came to see me about her sex life, which was in total disarray. Julie related that for twelve months she had not felt any sexual urges, and that when she had sex, it was merely to please her husband, who by all accounts was as virile as ever. During sex, Julie found that she experienced a burning pain and tightness in her vagina, which caused her to feel anxious and sweat profusely. Doctors use the term dyspareunia to describe painful sexual intercourse, and Julie's symptoms certainly fitted into this category. Julie also complained that stimulation of her clitoris was no longer pleasurable; indeed, she had noticed that her clitoris was shrinking and felt tender and fragile.

'I'm definitely not the sexpot I used to be,' Julie said, adding that she felt her husband was taking her lack of response personally, so that he was beginning to doubt his ability to be a passionate lover.

Examination of Julie's vagina showed it to be affected by a lack of sex hormones – it was pale in colour and its mucous membranes were thin, dry, and fragile. Her clitoris was very small, inflamed, and tender. Thankfully, her ovaries felt normal and she had no sign of prolapse of the vagina. A blood test revealed that Julie had started menopause, as her levels of oestrogen and testosterone were very low.

Julie decided that she wanted to try hormone replacement therapy to bring her hormonal levels back into the normal range. I reassured her that HRT would reverse the ageing changes that had occurred in the sexual areas of her anatomy.

I gave Julie an injection of a mixture of natural oestrogen and testosterone (called Primodian in Australia but unavailable in the UK), which restores the levels of the sex hormones oestrogen and testosterone in the body. Four weeks later Julie returned, saying, as

I knew she would, that she had found her former sexual persona and was now able to enjoy sex, lubricate after stimulation, and have satisfying orgasms. Her dyspareunia had vanished. She was also pleased that the oestrogen in the injection had made her shrinking breasts rounder and fuller.

Julie had enjoyed her mental and physical response to HRT and wanted to maintain the effect of the injection. I explained to her that the injection's effect would only last six to eight weeks and that to continue feeling the way she felt now, the most effective strategy would be to insert an implant of 100 mg of oestrogen and 100 mg of testosterone into the fat of her buttocks. Such an implant would last for approximately twelve months, and she could then have another implant. This idea appealed to Julie as she could not be bothered with tablets or patches in her busy lifestyle, which involved a lot of travel. Before inserting the implant, I warned Julie that the testosterone implant may cause a slight increase in facial pimples and hair, however for Julie this was a small price to pay. If you do not feel this way yourself, a smaller 50mg testosterone implant can be substituted and is less likely to cause these nuisance side-effects. Alternatively, an implant of oestrogen alone can be used, which will help greatly with your sex life, but to lesser degree than if you received both oestrogen and testosterone in your implant. Testosterone has the effects of increasing your libido (sex drive) and may cause slight enlargement of the clitoris. Some women choose to take testosterone initially in their long-term programme of HRT, others choose to use it intermittently, say once every few years, while many women feel it is not for them at all. Your sexual needs may change as you age and your HRT can be modified to blend in with this.

Many women find menopause to be a sexually fulfilling and exciting time because they are better able to relax once they are free of the fear of unwanted pregnancy. They also tend to be more in touch with and comfortable about their sexual needs and desires than they were earlier in life. Unfortunately, however, there are also many women – like Julie – who find that menopause has an unfavourable impact on their sex lives. There are a number of different changes that can occur during menopause that may cause sexual problems.

VAGINAL DRYNESS

Many of the sexual difficulties menopausal women experience are a direct result of declining levels of sex hormones. Among other things, deficiencies of the sex hormones oestrogen and testosterone often produce shrinkage and dryness of the vagina and vaginal lips (see Figure 17) and reduce sexual desire.

As discussed in Chapter 1, over half of all women at menopause and beyond are bothered by dryness of the vaginal tissues. This can lead to discomfort and even pain during sexual intercourse.

There are several different strategies that you can use, either singly or in combination, to overcome vaginal dryness and fragility. For a temporary lubricating action, you can use a bland jelly, such as K-Y jelly, or vitamin E cream, which also has a healing effect. These can be used before or during sexual intercourse, as needed. There are also over-the-counter products, such as Replens, that are formulated specifically for this condition and that, when used on an ongoing basis, supposedly afford longer-lasting relief. All of these products are available at pharmacies without a prescription.

To actually restore and strengthen the vagina and vulva, however, you need to use a hormonal cream or vaginal suppository, especially if your menopause was early or you want to resume sexual activity after a long period of abstinence. Hormonal creams and vaginal suppositories rejuvenate, thicken, and moisten the mucosal folds and lining of the vagina and the vaginal lips, and they improve blood circulation to the clitoral area, thus restoring the capacity for natural lubrication and orgasm. If you feel that your **vagina has shrunk and is too small for your partner's penis, this can be overcome by regularly massaging the inside and opening of the** vaginal walls using an oestrogen cream. Place some oestrogen cream on your fingers and rub it into the vaginal walls, gently stretching the walls apart and exerting gentle pressure backwards at the opening of the vagina. It is most comfortable to do this while lying down. It can be done gradually more and more each day. There is no need to stretch excessively and cause any discomfort. Ten minutes daily of this gentle massage and stretching is sufficient. Oestrogen creams and suppositories require a doctor's prescription, as they contain hormones; suitable brands are Premarin, Ovestin, and Dienoestrol. For some women, especially if the clitoris has become very small, the addition of testosterone to the vaginal oestrogen cream can make it much more effective than oestrogen cream alone in restoring sexual responsiveness. The clitoris is normally the size of an average pea (see Figure 17).

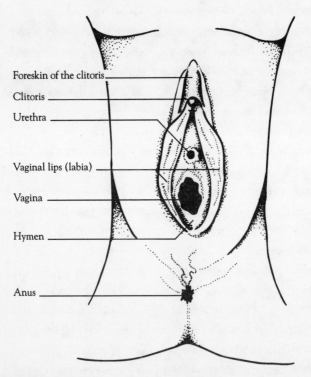

Foreskin of the clitoris

Clitoris

Urethra

Vaginal lips (labia)

Vagina

Hymen

Anus

Figure 17 **A woman's external sex organs**

You can ask your doctor to write a prescription for your pharmacist to mix you a special vaginal cream containing both oestrogen and testosterone. While the precise proportions of ingredients may vary somewhat depending on the individual's needs, a good basic formula is as follows:

- 40 per cent oestrogen cream (Premarin cream or the equivalent).
- 20 per cent testosterone (from three ampoules of injectable Primoteston Depot).
- 20 per cent petroleum jelly.
- 20 per cent Sorbolene and glycerine (made by mixing nine parts Sorbolene cream to one part glycerine).

You may massage your vagina, vulva, and clitoris with this cream every night for three to four weeks, after which time you should need to use it only twice a week. Some of my patients have told me that their hormonal creams or suppositories act like an aphrodisiac and make them feel more sexy!

POOR SEX DRIVE

If you are worried by a lack of sex drive, ask your doctor to do a blood test to measure your levels of the various hormones that are important determinants of libido and sexual well-being. It does not matter if you are already taking HRT, as some women on HRT still find that their sex life is poor. This could mean that your HRT needs adjusting.

The blood test should measure four things:

1 Follicle-stimulating hormone (FSH). If your FSH level is very high, say, above 50 milli-international units per millilitre (mIU/mL), then you should benefit from taking oestrogen. If you already take oestrogen, it may help to increase the dosage.
2 Oestradiol. This is the biochemical name for oestrogen. If the

level of oestradiol in your blood is consistently less than 200pmol/L, you may benefit from taking oestrogen; if you are already taking HRT, a larger dose or different form of oestrogen may help. If a woman taking oestrogen tablets has a very active liver, it may break down the oestrogen as soon as it is absorbed from the intestine and passes through the liver. In other words, the liver may weaken the effect of the oestrogen before it has a chance to work on your mind and sexual organs. If this is the case, you may find that you need increasing doses of oestrogen tablets to feel normal, and yet your blood oestrogen levels remain low. Increasing your dose of oral oestrogen may help, but, of course, one cannot go on increasing the dosage of oestrogen tablets indefinitely, as side-effect such as nausea, fluid retention, and breast swelling may result.

If your liver is very active and your oestrogen tablets are no longer relieving your symptoms, I suggest you ask your doctor about forms of oestrogen that bypass the liver – namely, patches, implants or injections – or take your oestrogen tablets vaginally. Some women find that they get better results if they insert their oestrogen tablets high into the vagina instead of taking them by mouth, because this allows the oestrogen to be absorbed directly into the bloodstream from the vagina and thus bypass the liver. Consequently, some women find that their libido and sexual responsiveness improve after transferring to a form of oestrogen replacement therapy that is not taken by mouth.

3. Sex hormone binding globulin (SHBG). This is a protein produced by the liver, and its function is to bind sex hormones such as oestrogen, progesterone, and testosterone and carry them around in the bloodstream. In much the same way that a car transports you along a freeway, SHBG transports your sex hormones along your blood vessels. While they are bound to SHBG, however, the sex hormones are not active in your body. Thus, if you have too much sex hormone binding globulin in

your blood, the majority of your sex hormones will be bound and inactive. Chances are that, as a result, you will feel not only sexless but tired and grumpy as well. On the other hand, if you have too little SHBG, this can result in acne or excess facial hair. Ideally, your SHBG level should fall somewhere in the middle of the normal range, which is 30 to 90nmol/L. In other words, it is undesirable to have either too little or too much SHBG.

I see many women who complain of having lost their sexuality, and in many cases I find that their blood tests reveal very high levels of SHBG. Why is this? Once again, you can blame the liver, and it is the oral forms of oestrogen that most stimulate the liver to produce increased amounts of SHBG. If your SHBG is high (90nmol/L or more), you may find that your sex life and general energy level improve if you transfer to a non-oral form of oestrogen such as patches, implants or injections, or if you take your oestrogen tablets via your vagina. If the oestrogen bypasses your liver in this way, the liver will be less stimulated to make SHBG and your levels of SHBG should start to fall.

If you have high levels of SHBG, a small dose of testosterone may also help as – don't forget – SHBG also binds the hormone testosterone, inactivating it. Testosterone is best given in the form of implants or injections, and can really bring the zing back into a tired sex life.

4 Androgens. These are also sometimes referred to as 'male hormones', but in fact women too require some of these masculinizing hormones in their bodies (albeit much less than men) to give them a healthy sex drive and for general mental and physical well-being. The tests that are useful are those that measure total testosterone, free testosterone, and free androgens. The free hormones are the ones that are not bound **by SHBG and are thus active in your body. If your doctor finds that your free testosterone and free androgen levels are very**

low, this can explain symptoms of fatigue and loss of sex drive, and these problems can easily be overcome by taking some testosterone in the form of implants or injections.

Testosterone has the effect of increasing libido and may cause slight enlargement of the clitoris, depending on the dosage taken. Some women choose to take testosterone as part of their long-term programme of HRT; others take it only initially or intermittently, say, once every four to six months. On the other hand, many women feel they do not need it at all. Your needs may change as you age, and your HRT can be modified to respond to this.

Poor libido can also be helped greatly by improving your diet and lifestyle. Avoid smoking and drinking excessive amounts of alcohol. Both of these can cause fatigue and reduce sexual response and performance.

The oestrogenic foods and herbs mentioned in Chapter 6 can increase your oestrogen levels naturally, so take these during times of a sexual low. The best herbs for increasing sex drive are damiana, dong quai, sarsaparilla, red clover, and black cohosh (see page 141–5). Soyabeans, soya sprouts and alfalfa sprouts, if eaten four to five times per week, will boost oestrogen levels so that you may start feeling quite sexy again! Also, take 2,000 to 3,000 milligrams of evening primrose oil, 500 milligrams of vitamin E, and 30 milligrams of zinc chelate daily to aid your adrenal gland in producing sex hormones.

How are your dreams? Are they lacking in sexual content? If so, try a combination of 500 milligrams of choline, 500 milligrams of pantothenic acid (vitamin B5), and 100 milligrams of vitamin B6 (pyridoxine) daily. This will boost your levels of the neurotransmitters serotonin and acetylcholine, which are involved in libido and sexual response. I see many husbands urgently writing this little combination down during my seminars on menopause!

INFLAMMATION AND INFECTION OF PELVIC TISSUE

In some menopausal women, recurrent vaginal and bladder inflammation and/or infections make them feel very tender and itchy, and most unsexy. These things occur partly because your sexual tissues are more vulnerable to infections and trauma without hormones. Hormone replacement therapy and vaginal creams can take care of this. If your vagina and vulva remain tender and inflamed and you continue to suffer bladder infections, urinary frequency, and burning, you need to boost your immune system with diet and nutritional supplements. To boost your immune system, I recommend the following:

- Drink two litres of purified or bottled water daily.
- Drink two to three glasses of raw vegetable juices daily.
- Avoid refined sugar, alcohol, caffeine, cigarettes, foods containing refined sugar, and yeast products (eat yeast-free bread).
- Eat plenty of raw vegetables and fruit.
- Take 3,000 milligrams of evening primrose oil daily.
- Take an antioxidant supplement containing vitamin A or beta-carotene, vitamin C, bioflavonoids, vitamin E, and selenium. Take a total of 10,000 international units of vitamin A (or 20 milligrams of beta-carotene), 5,000 milligrams of vitamin C with bioflavonoids, 500 international units of vitamin E, and 50 micrograms of selenium daily.
- Take 1,000 to 2,000 milligrams of garlic or odourless garlic capsules daily.
- Take *Lactobacillus acidophilus* capsules or powder, or eat acidophilus yoghurt daily.

These simple and safe strategies are extremely effective for overcoming recurrent infections or inflammation in the vagina and bladder, although they may take several months to bring relief. They are certainly safer than taking frequent courses of antibiotic drugs which, in the long term, only weaken your own immune system. Please see your doctor if symptoms persist.

POOR GENERAL HEALTH AND MEDICAL PROBLEMS

If you suffer from chronic fatigue, severe stress, or any recurrent painful condition, or if you feel generally unwell, you will probably have a reduced interest in sexual activity as a result. See Chapters 6 and 7 for valuable information to help you improve your general health. You should also discuss any chronic or recurring health problems, and their effects on your sex life, with your health care provider.

Women who smoke heavily often notice a big reduction in their sexual response as they age. This is because the phases of sexual excitement, lubrication, and orgasm are due to the congestion and swelling with blood of the erotic tissues in the clitoris, vulva, and vagina. Smoking damages the small blood vessels all over the body, including those in the vaginal area, so that they are less able to swell up with blood in response to sexual stimulation. Thus, your sexual response can be impaired by heavy smoking.

PRESCRIPTION MEDICATIONS

A wide range of drugs may affect sexual function, causing loss of libido, difficulty in becoming sexually aroused, and orgasmic dysfunction. The most common drugs that cause these symptoms are appetite suppressants, some muscle relaxants, some drugs used to treat epilepsy, some drugs to prevent headaches, some high blood pressure medications, some sedatives and anti-depressant drugs, some anti-ulcer drugs, and anti-male hormone drugs. Make sure you talk to your doctor about this before you begin taking a new medication, as you may be upset to find your sexual ability and desire lessened by the medication. There may be suitable alternative products that will not have this effect. New forms of many older drugs that have fewer side-effects and no adverse effects on libido are becoming available.

PROLAPSE

Menopausal women may develop certain physical problems that can cause their sex lives to deteriorate – namely, prolapse of the vagina, bladder, bowel, and/or uterus. The term *prolapse* means a loosening and falling down of tissues or organs due to stretching and the force of gravity with advancing years. Areas prone to prolapse include the uterus and the back wall of the vagina (see Figure 18). The front wall of the vagina may also prolapse. If it does, the bladder often prolapses with it, forming a swelling that can be seen when you cough. This combined bladder and vaginal prolapse is called a cystocele. Women with a cystocele often have problems with stress incontinence, meaning that when they cough, strain, or run, they pass urine involuntarily. If the back wall of the vagina prolapses, the lower bowel (the rectum) often prolapses down into it, forming a swelling that may fill with faeces, especially if you are constipated. This swelling is called a rectocele (see Figure 18).

If the uterus prolapses down into the vagina, a more solid swelling can be felt or seen and, in severe cases, the cervix protrudes outside of the vaginal opening. Women with uterine prolapse have usually had several children, or experienced difficult and prolonged labour.

It is easy to understand why, with any type of prolapse, sexual intercourse may be uncomfortable and perhaps a little embarrassing. Also, with prolapse, the vaginal and pelvic floor muscles are stretched to such a degree that both the woman and her partner may find the vagina is too big for either of them to feel very much during intercourse.

In moderate to severe cases of prolapse, a surgical vaginal repair is necessary. This can be done completely through incisions in the vagina. A vaginal repair will eliminate a cystocele or rectocele, reduce or cure stress incontinence, and make your vagina a normal snug size so that sexual intercourse once again becomes enjoyable.

If your uterus has prolapsed down into the vagina, you will probably have a dull, dragging discomfort in your pelvic and vaginal areas. Your doctor will probably offer you a choice of surgical treatments: either having your uterus removed (hysterectomy) or having the uterine ligaments repaired so that the uterus is no longer prolapsed. In most cases of uterine prolapse, the uterus can be removed through the vagina at the same time a vaginal repair (if needed) is done, and this has the advantage that no abdominal incisions are required. Your gynaecologist should explain the various surgical techniques to you in full before you decide which is best for you.

In milder cases of vaginal prolapse, Kegel's exercises, done to strengthen muscles in the vagina and pelvic floor, are often effective. These can be done in two ways:

1 Tighten and squeeze your vagina and rectum by drawing your muscles inwards and upwards. Hold this position for five to ten seconds, then relax. Repeat the exercise as many times as possible, gradually working up to 100 to 200 repetitions each day. This exercise can be done anywhere – while driving, sitting on the train, watching television, etc. – and no one can see you doing it.
2 While passing urine, practise starting and stopping the flow of urine as many times as you can. This exercise will help women with stress incontinence.

If your prolapse is not too bad and you practise these exercises daily, after three to four months you may find that surgical repair is no longer needed. As an added bonus you will find that your muscular control of the vagina and pelvic floor during sex has improved, thus giving greater sexual pleasure to both you and your partner.

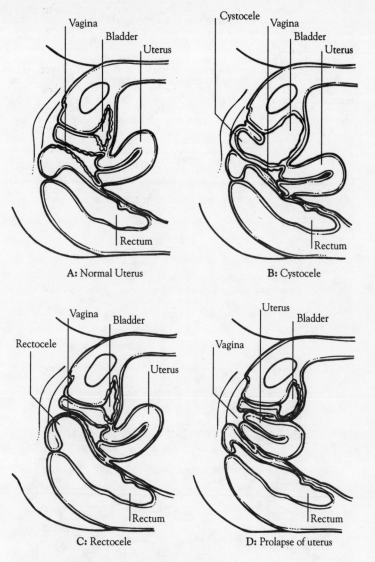

Figure 18 **Different types of prolapse**

After menopause, the ligaments and muscles that support a woman's reproductive organs in their normal position (A) can weaken. This can result in a prolapse of the uterus (D), in which the uterus falls downward into the vagina, or of the vagina. If the front wall of the vagina prolapses, the bladder may prolapse with it, creating a cystocele (B). If the back wall or the vagina prolapses, the rectum may prolapse down into the vagina, forming a rectocele (C).

YOUR STATE OF MIND

Some women find that menopause is a time of sexual liberation, and that their sex lives become better than ever. This may be because they no longer have to worry about pregnancy and contraception, and also because they have more time, space, and privacy to have a relaxed sex life. By the age of forty, most women have become aware of their sexual needs and preferences and feel comfortable about telling their partners how to please them. This is a wonderful thing, and very important for the sexual pleasure of both partners. If you find you are not able to express fully your sexual needs to your partner, it is very important that you try to improve communication. If you are not successful doing this on your own, it may be helpful to seek counselling.

Patients on hormone therapy may start to behave in a more provocative way!

Whether you are married or have an older or younger lover, menopause and the years surrounding it can bring you great sexual satisfaction. Many women tell me that their sex lives improve with age – 'just like a good wine!' they say – and this is important to most women. So I want to reassure you that there is sex after menopause, and it can be very beautiful, gentle, and relaxing. The need to perform or be orgasmic mellows with age, and many couples find that sex becomes more emotional and affectionate.

On the other hand, if you would rather go to bed with a hot water bottle and a good book, that's normal, too. Many women find that once their sex hormones no longer surge, they feel a more intense urge to study, be creative, or take up new pursuits. For some women, it's great no longer to have men treating them as 'sex objects', and they feel quite at ease saying, 'Not tonight, darling, I've got to finish something else.' The important thing is to enjoy being yourself, at both sexy times and tranquil times, during this unique phase of life.

CHAPTER NINE

MALE MENOPAUSE – FACT OR FICTION?

This chapter is designed for both you and your partner, especially if he has a midlife crisis. We have all heard the phrase, whether used seriously or jokingly, but is there really such a thing as 'male menopause'? In this chapter I will sort out the fact from the fiction. What you learn may surprise you.

The *menopause* literally means the cessation of menstrual bleeding. In females, this signifies that the biological clock has stopped and infertility has set in, accompanied by dramatic hormonal changes. So technically, the word *menopause* obviously cannot apply to men. Yet it is indeed a fact that men also are vulnerable to fundamental emotional, mental, and physical changes at about fifty years of age and beyond.

HORMONAL CHANGES IN MEN

The production of testosterone by the testicles is at its peak during a man's twenties and thirties. Thereafter, a slow decline occurs. This decline becomes more noticeable after the age of thirty. However, there are large variations among individuals; some men at fifty produce such low levels of testosterone that they no longer feel any inclination to have a sex life, whereas others have high testosterone levels and are still vigorous at eighty. As you read this, you are probably wondering how your partner (or you, if you are a male) can be one of the lucky ones. The ability to produce testosterone is partly genetic, so in many cases it's 'like father like son'. Lifestyle also plays a role. Men who smoke and/or drink alcohol excessively have lower levels of testosterone in their blood than those who do not. Furthermore, as a man ages, not only does the production of testosterone diminish, but so does the ability of his tissues and cells to respond to testosterone.

Finding out if a man's testosterone level is down is a matter of a simple blood test. For men, the amount of testosterone in the blood is 11–37 nmol/L. A deficiency of testosterone is obvious if the blood level falls below 10 nmol/L. This would be further corroborated if the level of a pituitary hormone called luteinizing hormone (LH) is high, as this would indicate that the pituitary gland is trying to stimulate the sluggish testicles. This blood test may be repeated on three separate occasions, at eight-week intervals, to demonstrate a consistent deficiency of testosterone.

Symptoms of Testosterone Deficiency

Testosterone deficiency shows up in a number of ways, including:

- Fatigue, reduced libido, and behavioural changes.
- Atrophy (shrinkage) of the muscles, testicles and penis, and softening of the testicles.
- A reduced rate of growth of facial and body hair.
- A reduction in virility and the ability to achieve orgasm (in severe cases, impotence).

A man in midlife who previously had high levels of testosterone may find himself experiencing subtle mental and physical changes as a result of decreasing testosterone levels, even though blood tests reveal that his testosterone levels are still within the normal range. This is because even though technically normal, his testosterone level is much lower than it used to be, and he is sensitive to the decreasing level.

Subtle changes resulting from decreasing testosterone production may range from depression and loss of confidence to a loss of drive and a decline in aggression and competitiveness in all spheres. The warrior man may find himself becoming a bit of a mouse. If such a man gets himself to the doctor, he may be told that all this is symptomatic of a psychological midlife crisis, especially if a full check-up fails to reveal any medical problems. He may be told that this crisis is due to a plateau in his career, looming retirement, unrealized ambitions, getting older, stress, or just overdoing it. Consequently, he may be offered a course of anti-depressants, sedatives, or tranquillizers, and referred for counselling to assuage his growing self-doubts. Men tend to be more reluctant than women to accept a course of such therapy; many prefer to numb their anxieties at the bar with their buddies. Unfortunately, alcohol ingestion, if it becomes regular or excessive, often further reduces a man's production of testosterone, making his mental and physical balance worse.

It is vital to check the possibility of a hormonal contribution if a man in midlife experiences progressive symptoms of depression, loss of ambition, or loss of libido. And if tests suggest a deficiency of testosterone, hormone replacement therapy may be of help and a short course of testosterone replacement can be tried.

HORMONE REPLACEMENT THERAPY FOR MEN

The first semblance of HRT was actually used on a man, not a woman. In 1889, a then-famous neurophysiologist named Charles-Edward Brown-Sequard treated himself with an extract of animal testicles, which produced, in his own words, 'a return of vigour, youthful appetites and desires'. Today, hormone replacement therapy for men is available and can be taken in different forms, including oral androgens, androgen injections and implants. Nowadays it is not unusual for a 'menopausal' male to receive hormonal treatment, although the percentage of men who do is dramatically lower than the percentage of women who try HRT for menopause.

ORAL ANDROGENS

The word *androgen* is the medical term for the so-called male hormones – those sex hormones that have masculinizing effects on the body. Androgens may be taken on a regular basis in tablet form. Two common androgens available in tablet form are testosterone undecanoate (Restandol) or mesterolone (Pro-Viron). There is a possible link between methyltestosterone and liver cancer, however, and oral androgens can produce nausea if taken in large doses.

All in all, oral androgens are variable in their effect. Some men with severe testosterone deficiency complain that oral testosterone does not help them. In such cases, testosterone injections or implants may be much more effective.

ANDROGEN INJECTIONS

If a man is considering a short-term trial of HRT, there is probably no more definitive way of assessing its benefits than a three- or four-month course of monthly injections of androgen. If a deficiency of testosterone is responsible for the mental, physical, and sexual fatigue of middle age, an androgen injection should greatly reduce, if not abolish, these symptoms within one to two weeks. This brings a great sense of relief. In addition to alleviating symptoms, androgen injections can produce a feeling of great energy and vitality, and can be a superb anti-depressant.

Suitable injectable androgens are testosterone oenanthate (Primoteston Depot) or testosterone propionate (Sustanon). Either of these can be taken as a deep intramuscular injection into the buttocks, usually once a month for three to four months. A follow-up appointment with the doctor should be made for three months after the final injection, by which time the effect of the injections should no longer be apparent. During this consultation, the decision either to abandon testosterone therapy or to continue with it for the long term can be made. If a patient decides to continue with the treatment for several years, the most effective way to deliver testosterone to the tissues would be via a hormone implant.

ANDROGEN IMPLANTS

Each implant contains 200 mg of testosterone and if three of these are inserted at once, they will provide good blood levels of testosterone for six months. The implants are buried into the fat of the abdominal wall or buttocks. Most men find these implants very effective and free of side-effects. This is understandable, as the testosterone is absorbed from the implant directly into the blood, bypassing the liver, and is carried to the receptive tissues and organs (see Figure 14, page 90).

SIDE-EFFECTS OF ANDROGEN REPLACEMENT THERAPY

If a man takes testosterone in any form – whether tablets or injections – on a long-term basis, the course of the therapy must be carefully supervised by a doctor. Testosterone replacement therapy taken over several to many years may cause side-effects. The tablet forms are probably more likely to do this than are the other forms. Ideally, the lowest possible dose of testosterone that maintains a good quality of mental, physical, and sexual well-being should be used.

Testosterone replacement therapy can increase the size of the prostate gland. The prostate gland is a small, somewhat pyramid-shaped organ that is situated at the neck of the bladder and secretes fluid to add to the sperm during ejaculation. If the prostate gland becomes enlarged, a man may experience difficulty in passing urine, with such symptoms as difficulty in beginning urination, dribbling after passing urine, slowness and delay in completing urination, and urinary frequency. If these problems persist, surgical removal of the prostate gland may be required.

There are other potential consequences of testosterone replacement therapy as well. Long-term testosterone replacement therapy may increase the risk of cancer of the prostate gland. If testosterone doses are excessive, they may have an unfavourable effect on blood cholesterol patterns, increasing the risk of cardiovascular disease. Excessive doses may also produce polycythemia (an abnormally high level of red blood cells) and significant weight gain.

Overall, however, testosterone replacement therapy – while not without risk – is safe and can be of tremendous value, provided it is prescribed by an expert in the field and followed by annual check-ups from a urologist.

CAN 'MALE MENOPAUSE' CAUSE IMPOTENCE?

Minor degrees of testosterone deficiency do not cause impotence. A man's level of testosterone deficiency would need to be marked before inability to achieve erection and orgasm occurred. Most men who consult a doctor about impotence in midlife do *not* have a significant testosterone deficiency.

Other factors, such as general fitness, cardiovascular status, long-term abuse of cigarettes and alcohol, the consumption of certain medications, stress, and loss of confidence are more likely causes of impotence, especially if two or more of these factors occur in combination. Most men who suffer from impotence have a functional disorder of the 'spongy' erectile tissue in the penis. This erectile tissue is called the *corpus cavernosum*, and during a normal erection, it becomes congested with blood. If this congestion does not occur, the penis remains small and soft. New treatments available for this problem are vasoactive drugs such as alprostadil (also known as prostaglandin E, and sold under the name Caverject) that can be self-injected into the erectile tissue of the penis when required. These injections enable a man to regain control of his erections, although by artificial means. Most users of this method are very satisfied. If this fails, penile implants can be successful. For more detailed information about male impotence, I recommend the excellent and comprehensive book *It's Up to You* by Warwick Williams.[1]

OESTROGEN THERAPY FOR MEN

It used to be thought that the hormone oestrogen exerted effects only on female sexual organs, such as the vagina, uterus and breasts. We now know that oestrogen exerts profound and widespread effects upon many other tissues, such as the brain, liver, bones, joints, skin, heart, and arteries. In particular, oestrogen has a very favourable effect on blood cholesterol, as it helps the enzymes that break down cholesterol and thus reduces the chances of the blood vessels becoming blocked with plaque. In the long term, oestrogen helps to reduce diseases of the heart and blood vessels.

This observation has led some of our modern-day scientists to come up with the hypothesis that if we give natural oestrogen to males, we may be able to reduce their current high rate of cardiovascular disease. Indeed there are now clinical trials underway to see if giving natural oestrogen to men between the ages of thirty and sixty will reduce their cholesterol levels and incidence of heart attacks. Oestrogen may also reduce the incidence of cancer of the prostate gland, so there are several ways in which oestrogen might give men an extra ten years or so of life.

All is not roses, however. Oestrogen is a potent feminizing hormone, so it is likely to have some undesirable side-effects for the male of the species. These could include breast tenderness, loss of sex drive, impotence, and reduced sperm production.

NUTRITIONAL STRATEGIES FOR 'MALE MENOPAUSE'

Diet and lifestyle are supremely important for the man who finds himself with reduced mental and sexual performance during midlife.

Exercise is vitally important. However, given the current high rate of cardiovascular disease among men, I believe all men should undergo a cardiac stress test (exercise ECG) before initiating an increase in their exercise programme. A good age to have a cardiac stress test is forty to fifty – or even younger if there is a poor family history.

There are also some specific vitamins, minerals, herbs, and dietary supplements that can improve the functioning of the endocrine system, and in particular that of the testicles. Among the most important supplements for men in midlife are vitamin E, magnesium, zinc, ginseng, royal jelly, and the entire vitamin B complex. Table 11 provides an overview of these supplements, their function, and recommended doses.

VITAMIN E

I believe that all middle-aged men should take 500 international units of vitamin E (d-alpha-tocopheral) daily. Vitamin E is a superb antioxidant that is especially active in the *intima* (the inner layer of the arteries) and reduces artherosclerosis (hardening of the arteries) and heart disease. To remain sexually active and virile, you need healthy blood vessels to supply blood to the pelvic area.

MAGNESIUM

Although sodium is the dominant mineral in today's oceans, the primordial oceans of the earth were rich in magnesium and potassium. The cytoplasm (intracellular fluid) in our bodies still resembles the 'primordial soup' from which all forms of life arose. Our intracellular fluid is rich in the minerals magnesium and potassium, and our body works hard to maintain this state. Magnesium is found mainly in the bones, the muscles, and the fluid within our cells. It is vital for every important biological reaction, including the synthesis of protein and of genetic material, the metabolism of glucose, and the release of cellular energy.

Adequate magnesium is vital for a healthy cardiovascular system because it regulates nerve conduction, vascular tone, and the electrical stability of muscle cells, and it is essential for maintaining the integrity of cell membranes. Marginal magnesium deficiency is very common in many men, especially diabetics, regular drinkers, poor eaters, and those who exercise regularly and strenuously. Magnesium supplementation may reduce ischaemic heart disease, cardiac arrhythmias, and cardiomyopathy. Good food sources of magnesium include seafoods, green vegetables, nuts, and low-fat dairy products. Recommended supplemental doses range from 250 to 800 milligrams of magnesium amino acid chelate daily.

ZINC

A daily 50-milligram zinc chelate supplement is most worthwhile for men. There is evidence that most of us become increasingly prone to zinc deficiency with age, and even in developed countries many men are at risk of marginal zinc deficiencies.

Zinc can increase male potency and libido, and may reduce prostate problems such as prostatitis (inflammation) and hypertrophy (enlargement). Also, gentlemen, it can reduce hair loss and aches and pains in the muscles and joints. However, you should be careful not to exceed the recommended dosage, as excessive amounts of zinc can cause stomach upset. Zinc is best taken intermittently– for example, three months on, three months off.

GINSENG

Ginseng is probably the most ancient and famous medicinal herb on earth. Its use in Chinese medicine dates back more than 4,000 years. Soviet scientists began investigating ginseng in the mid-twentieth century, and found that it increased the body's resistance to a wide range of adverse factors.

There are two types of ginseng, Siberian (botanical name *Eleutherococcus senticosus*) and American (*Panax quinquefolius*). Better results seem to come from Siberian ginseng. Russian researchers claim that ginseng can boost immunity, inhibit cancer, and increase energy and stamina. Ginseng also enjoys a reputation as a 'glandular tonic' for men, meaning that it improves testicular functions.

Recommended doses range from 1,000 to 4,000 milligrams daily. However, ginseng should not be used by people with very high blood pressure (over 180/100).

ROYAL JELLY

This is the diet of the queen bee, and it is a potent mixture of pollen and special secretions from the glands of worker bees. It is a rich natural food containing vitamins, minerals, amino acids, and other nutrients. It is especially rich in choline, one of the precursors of acetylcholine, which is a neurotransmitter involved in sexual response and performance. Royal jelly has been used for centuries by the Chinese for its energy-boosting properties.

VITAMIN B COMPLEX

The B vitamins are essential for the normal functioning of the brain and peripheral nerves and thus for a healthy sex life. In particular, vitamin B6 (pyridoxine), vitamin B5 (pantothenic acid), and choline are needed for the manufacture of the neurotransmitters serotonin and acetylcholine. These neurotransmitters are vital for libido and for sexual performance and enjoyment. Acetylcholine is a memory-enhancing neurotransmitter and a balancer of the nervous system.

Many men and women, especially regular drinkers, are lacking some of the B vitamins, and would benefit by taking a vitamin B supplement. A good B complex tablet should contain vitamins B1 (thiamine), B2 (riboflavin), B3 (niacin), B5 (pantothenic acid), B6 (pyridoxine), B12 (cyancobalamin), and choline and should be taken on a daily basis.

MALE MIDLIFE CRISIS

We know that, technically speaking, men cannot go through a literal menopause. However, for many men midlife brings significant hormonal, physical, and psychological changes. Put these all together in a melting pot and you may very well have the ingredients for a male midlife crisis. This is undoubtedly one of the reasons why divorce rates soar at this time of life, and many women get the shock of their lives. Many women are left alone in their 'empty nests' as their husbands flee the familiar domestic scene. Conversely, the male not infrequently gets the 'nesting syndrome' and spreads his wings with a younger woman, finding that her youthfulness rekindles his feeling of manliness and passion, and feeling that life is beginning all over again. Of course, the women they leave behind can also get the 'nesting syndrome' and run off with younger men. I see quite a few older women doing this and find it an interesting social phenomenon. And after all, women in general live longer than men do – six years longer overall, and nine to ten years for women who take natural oestrogen at menopause – so to help avoid loneliness in old age, a man ten years younger could probably fit the bill very nicely.

Usually, however, such situations are very emotional and can be extremely traumatic in both the short and long term. Yet many of them could probably be averted if men received more information and supportive counselling, especially together with their wives, at this time in their lives. In some cases, the timely use of testosterone replacement therapy, even if only on a temporary basis, can put the sparkle back into a long-term sexual relationship.

A male who finds himself with symptoms of male menopause during midlife can be helped greatly either by hormone replacement therapy or by nutritional medicine and lifestyle changes. Yet many men feel ashamed to admit that they have lost their virility and prior energy and do not seek help. They either assume that no help is available, or they believe that it is

TABLE 11

MALE MENOPAUSE KIT

There are a number of dietary supplements that can be extremely helpful for men in midlife. The following table outlines a suggested daily programme of vitamins, mineral, and herbal supplements a man can use to improve his overall health and well-being.

SUPPLEMENT	DAILY DOSE	ACTIONS
Vitamin E	500 IU	As an antioxidant, vitamin E protects cell structures and reduces oxidative damage to the linings of blood vessels. Vitamin E also increases the efficiency of oxygen utilization by cardiac muscle and improves testicular function.
Minerals Magnesium Zinc Selenium Manganese	500 mg 50 mg 50 mcg 5mg	These minerals are antioxidants and work synergistically as catalysts for enzyme systems, increasing metabolic efficiency. Magnesium also improves cardiac function; zinc is helpful for symptoms of an enlarged prostate.
Ginseng and royal jelly	2,000–4,000mg each	These are ancient 'glandular tonics' used by Chinese and Russian civilizations. They boost energy and immunity.
Balanced vitamin B complex containing: B1 (thiamine) B2 (riboflavin) B3 (niacin) B5 (pantothenic acid) B6 (pyridoxine) B12 (cyancobalamin) Choline	1 tablet or capsule	The B vitamins are necessary for the efficient functioning of the central and peripheral nervous system. They are especially important for persons who are under stress or who consume excessive amounts of alcohol.
Evening primrose oil	3,000 mg	A good source of essential fatty acids, which improve the production and release of hormones (see page 171)

unacceptable to complain of such symptoms lest they be seen as old or unmanly.

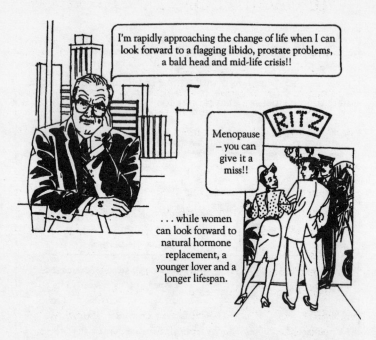

I'm rapidly approaching the change of life when I can look forward to a flagging libido, prostate problems, a bald head and mid-life crisis!!

Menopause – you can give it a miss!!

. . . while women can look forward to natural hormone replacement, a younger lover and a longer lifespan.

The female menopause is 'out of the closet' today, and women feel comfortable talking about their experiences and expressing their needs. Men should follow suit, and not worry about fitting the old fashioned stereotype of the macho male who never has (or at least never discusses) any problems or difficulties. Besides, it can be more character-building to 'open up' and confront one's problems, and to acknowledge the need to change. Men needn't worry that this will make them less manly or attractive, indeed, many women tell me that they prefer the kind of men we call 'snags' – 'sensitive new-age guys'.

Chapter ten

In Summary - A Farewell Message from the Author

When you arrive at menopause, there is no reason to fear a change of life for the worse. If you are well informed and aware of all your options, you have the tools to maintain, and even improve, your quality and enjoyment of life. In fact, there is some evidence suggesting that the better informed you are, the less likely you are to suffer in the first place.[1]

Menopause is a time of learning and self-appraisal. It is a time when you can take control of your life and shape its destiny. Above all, it is a time for taking pleasure in being a woman in your own unique style. And today, you have the opportunity to take advantage of the powerful benefits of preventative, nutritional, and herbal medicine; natural hormone replacement therapy; and an anti-ageing plan, to help ease your transition. You can have confidence in yourself and your decisions, which should give you the persistence necessary to obtain the best care and treatment available. Whatever you choose, be it 'designer HRT', orthodox medicine, nutritional or herbal medicine, Mother Nature, or a combination of any of these, you will be able to overcome any menopausal problems you may experience with accurate knowledge and a positive attitude.

You may go through occasional rough patches as you feel and see deep changes taking place in yourself. I hope that this handbook can serve you as a strong and meaningful lifeline at these times. Remember that I am feeling and understanding these changes with you, as are many of your sisters on this planet. If we gain inspiration, hope, and love from each other, something very precious will have been achieved.

I have written this because you and other women have inspired and taught me so much, and I know that we can continue to inspire and teach each other for many years. I hope it helps you to enjoy menopausal years and beyond. As far as I can see, this time of life can be the best ever!

Some Thoughts at Menopause

I have some lines in my face from fifty years of life.
They tell me of years in the sun, of sorrows and joys.
They tell me of time.
They tell me I have lived and that I am still alive.
They can't be erased. They can be softened...
Do I long to be the smooth-skinned , freckle-faced kid I once was?
No. I long for the same thing today that I longed for then:
to be the best I am able to be.[2]

In conclusion, I sincerely hope that you enjoyed this book and that you have found it useful in your own day-to-day life. There is so much to learn about our physical and mental well-being! Please feel free to write to me to give me feedback on this book or to make further enquiries.

My postal address is:

PO Box 217
Paddington
NSW 2021
Australia
or contact me via my e-mail address:
doctor-cabot@msn.com

NOTES

Chapter 1 Menopause in a Nutshell

1   J.W. Studd et al., 'Oestradiol and Testosterone Implants', *British Journal of Obstetrics and Gynaecology* 84 (1977): 314–15.

Chapter 2 The Long-Term Consequences of Oestrogen Deficiency

1   M.J. Stampfer, G.A. Colditz, et al., 'Postmenopausal Estrogen Therapy and Cardiovascular Disease', *New England Journal of Medicine* 325 (11) (12 September 1991): 756–62.

2   Ibid.

3   R. Bergstrom, M. Falkeborn, I. Persson, et al., 'Hormone Replacement Therapy and the Risk of Stroke: Follow-up of a Population-based Cohort in Sweden', *Archives of Internal Medicine* 153 (10) (24 May 1993): 1201–9.

4   Brian Henderson, 'An Epidemiological Evaluation of the Risks and Benefits of HRT', in *Proceedings of the Inaugural Scientific Meeting of the Australian Menopause Society* (Brisbane, Australia: Australian Menopause Society September 1989).

5   Ibid.

6   Stampfer, Colditz, et al., 'Postmenopausal Estrogen Therapy and Cardiovascular Disease'.

7   F.S. Kaplan, 'Osteoporosis: Pathophysiology and Prevention', in *Clinical Symposia*, Vol. 39 (1) (Ciba-Geigy Corporation, 1987), 1–32.

8   R.W. Smith, W.R. Eyler, and R.C. Mellingen, 'On the Incidence of Senile Osteoporosis', *Annals of Internal Medicine* 52 (1960): 773–6.

9   N.S. Weiss et al., 'Decreased Risk of Fractures of the Hip and Lower Forearm With Postmenopausal Use of Estrogen' *New England Journal of Medicine* 303 (1980): 1195–8.

10 Nelson B. Watts et al., 'Intermittent Cyclical Etidrontate Treatment of Postmenopausal Osteoporosis', *New England Journal of Medicine* 323 (12 July 1990): 73–9.

11 M.W. Tilyard et al., 'Treatment of Postmenopausal Osteoporosis With Calcitriol or Calcium', *New England Journal of Medicine* 326 (1992): 357–62.

Chapter 4 Everything You Will Ever Need to Know About HRT

1   Alvin H. Follinstad, MD, 'Oestriol. The Forgetten Oestrogen.' *Journal of the American Medical Association* Vol. 239, No. 1, 2 January 1978.

2   J.C. Stevenson et al., 'Effects of Transdermal Versus Oral Hormone Replacement Therapy on Bone Density in Spine and Proximal Femur in Postmenopausal Women', *Lancet* 336 No. II (1990): 265–9.

3   Linda Cordoza et al., 'The Effects of Subcutaneous Hormone Implants During the Climacteric', *Maturitas* 5 (1984): 177–84.

4   J.W. Studd et al., 'Oestradiol and Testosterone Implants', *British Journal of Obstetrics and Gynaecology* 84 (1977): 314–15.

Chapter 5 The Most-asked Questions about Menopause

1   Sandra Cabot, *The Body-Shaping Diet* (London: Boxtree, 1996).

2   R.D. Gambrell, Jr, 'Oestrogen-Progestogen Replacement and Cancer Risk',

Hospital Practice 15 (1990): 81–100.

3   B.K. Armstrong, 'Oestrogen Therapy – Boom or Bane?' *Medical Journal of Australia* 148 (1988): 213–4.

4   K.K. Steinberg et al., 'A Meta-analysis of the Effect of Estrogen Replacement Therapy on the Risk of Breast Cancer', *Journal of the American Medical Association* 265 (1991): 1985–90.

5   Ibid.

6   'The Use of Oestrogens and Progestins and the Risk of Breast Cancer in Postmenopausal Women', *New England Journal of Medicine*, Vol. 332, No. 24. 15 June 1995.

7   A.H. MacLennan, for the Australian Menopause Society, 'Consensus Statement. Hormone Replacement Therapy and the Menopause', *Medical Journal of Australia* 155 (1991): 43–4.

Chapter 6 Naturopathic Medicine for Menopause

1   K.D.R. Setchell et al., 'Non-steroidal Estrogens of Dietary Origin: Possible Roles in Hormone-Dependent Disease', *American Journal of Clinical Nutrition* 40 (September 1984): 569–78. H. Adlercreutz, T. Fotsis, et al., 'Determination of Urinary Lignans and Phytoestrogen Metabolites', *Journal of Steroid Biochemistry* 25 (5B) (November 1986): 791–7.

2   Barbara Evans, *Life Change* (London: Pan Books, 1979), 38.

3   R. Buist, 'The Role of Nutrients in the Prevention of Heart Disease', report to the seminar 'Nutrition in Disease Prevention', Sydney, Australia, Australian Council for Responsible Nutrition, 9 March 1992.

4   Ibid.

Chapter 7 Slowing Down the Ageing Process

1   Ruth Cilento, *Heal Cancer* (Australia: Hill of Content, 1993); Lewis Harrison, *Making Fats and Oils Work for You* (Garden City Park, NY: Avery Publishing Group, 1990).

2   Daniel Rudman et al., 'Effects of Human Growth Hormone in Men over 60 Years Old', *New England Journal of Medicine* 323 (1) (5 July 1990): 1–6.

3   Ibid.

Chapter 9 Male Menopause – Fact or Fiction?

1   Warwick Williams, *It's Up to You* (Sydney, Australia: Williams & Wilkins, 1985).

Chapter 10 In Summary – A Farewell Message from the Author

1   Barbara Evans, *Life Change* (London: Pan Books, 1979), 38.

2   Kaylan Pickford, *Always a Woman* (New York: Bantam Books, 1982).

GLOSSARY

Adipose tissue Fatty tissue.

Adrenal glands Two small glands situated on top of the kidneys that secrete various hormones, including adrenaline, cortisone, and sex hormones.

Agoraphobia Abnormal fear of open spaces. A person with severe agoraphobia will find it difficult or impossible to leave his or her home.

Anabolic steroids Synthetic hormones that stimulate the growth of bone muscle and have masculinizing effects on the body.

Androgen Sex hormones that promote the development of masculine characteristics, such as facial and body hair.

Antioxidant A substance that protects cellular structures against oxidative damage. Well-known antioxidants include vitamins A, C, and E, beta-carotene, the minerals zinc and selenium, and the enzyme superoxide dismutase (SOD).

Atrophy Wasting or thinning of tissues or organs.

Autoimmune disease Any of the group of diseases produced by an imbalance or malfunction of the immune system that causes the immune system to attack and inflame the body's own tissues and organs.

Cancer A type of disease characterized by the rapid multiplication of abnormal cells, resulting in a malignant growth, or tumour, that may spread to and invade distant body parts.

Cancer chemotherapy The administration of highly toxic chemical drugs into the body for the purpose of killing cancer cells.

Cardiovascular disease Any disease of the circulatory system, which comprises the heart and blood vessels.

Cervical smear A test in which cells are gently scraped from the cervix and smeared on to a glass slide for examination under a microscope. It is a screening test for cancer of the cervix.

Cholesterol A steroid classified as a lipid that is a constituent of all animal cells. High blood cholesterol levels increase the risk of cardiovascular disease. Dietary cholesterol is found in fats and oils of animal origin and in coconut oil.

Circulation The recurrent movement of the blood through the various blood vessels of the body.

Collagen A fibrous protein that gives elasticity and strength to the skin, bones, cartilage, and connective tissues.

Curettage The procedure of surgically scraping a body cavity (such as the uterus) to remove tissue, blood, or abnormal growths.

Deficiency Lack or insufficiency of an essential substance.

Dowager's hump A forward-facing curve on the upper spine, below the neck that forms as a result of compression of the spinal vertebrae.

Endocrine system The network of ductless glands that manufacture and secrete hormones into the bloodstream, affecting the functioning of distant organs and tissues.

Endocrinology The study and treatment of disorders of the glands and the hormones they secrete.

Endometrial ablation A surgical procedure in which the inner lining of the uterus is destroyed by means of radio waves or a laser beam.

Endometriosis A disorder in which the endometrial cells, which are normally confined inside the uterine cavity, are scattered about outside the uterus, in the abdomen, and/or in the pelvic cavity. It usually results in pain, possibly severe, during menstruation.

Endometrium The mucous membrane forming the inner layer or lining of the uterus.

Enzyme Any of the proteins that catalyse or facilitate chemical reactions in cells. They are necessary to break down, or metabolize, nutrients, drugs, and hormones.

Epidemiologist A specialist who deals with the spread of diseases among populations.

Essential fatty acids Fatty acids necessary for cellular metabolism that cannot be produced by the body but must be supplied in the diet. Suitable sources are evening primrose oil, fish oil, and various seeds and nuts.

Fallopian tubes The small tubes connected to the sides of the uterus, and in which fertilization occurs.

Fibroids Non-cancerous growths in the uterus that consist of muscle and fibrous tissue.

Follicle-stimulating hormone (FSH) A hormone secreted by the pituitary gland that acts on the ovary, causing it to stimulate the development (ripening) or follicles (eggs). These follicles produce oestrogen.

Frigidity Sexual unresponsiveness in a woman.

Genetic engineering Man-made alteration in the genetic structure of cells, usually done for breeding purposes, to eradicate diseases, or to enable cells to synthesize chemicals or hormones.

Gland *See* Endocrine system.

Hereditary The quality of being passed through the genes from the parents to their offspring, as characteristics or diseases.

Hormone Any of the chemicals that are produced by various glands in the body and transported in the blood to affect distant cells and organs.

Hormone replacement therapy (HRT) The administration of hormonal preparations (natural or synthetic) to make up for the decline of natural hormone production by various glands.

Hypertension High blood pressure.

Hypothalamus A major control centre of the brain that regulates temperature, appetite, thirst, and the function of hormonal glands. It is situated at the base of the brain and is directly connected to the pituitary gland.

Hysterectomy Surgical removal of the uterus.

Implant A chemical substance or object that is surgically implanted into a part of the body.

In vitro fertilization (IVF) Fertilization of the egg by the sperm outside the body, in a laboratory environment.

Incontinence The inability to restrain or control the discharge of urine or faeces.

Inflammation A condition characterized by swelling, redness, heat, and pain in any tissue. Inflammation may occur as a result of trauma, irritation, infection, or imbalances in immune function.

Insomnia The inability to sleep.

Libido Sexual desire.

Menopause The final cessation of menstruation; the last menstrual period.

Menstruation The cyclic (usually monthly) discharge of blood from the non-pregnant uterus; also called the menstrual period.

Metabolism The complex of chemical processes utilizing the raw materials of nutrients, oxygen, and vitamins, along with enzymes, to produce energy for body functions.

Glossary

Minerals A group of inorganic substances that are essential for normal cellular metabolism and the maintenance of life.

Mucous membrane A lubricating membrane lining an internal surface or an organ such as the intestines or genito-urinary canal.

Naturopathic medicine An approach to health care that emphasizes the prevention and treatment of illnesses with naturally occurring substances such as juices, vitamins, minerals, herbs, etc.

Oestradiol A natural oestrogen found in the blood. It is the most potent of all the natural oestrogens.

Oestrogen A sex hormone secreted primarily by the ovary that is responsible for female characteristics, such as the development of breasts and feminine curves, as well as for menstruation.

Oestrogen receptors Physical structures on the cell membranes that attract oestrogen and respond to its effects.

Oestrone A natural oestrogen found in the blood.

Osteoporosis A disorder characterized by loss of bone mass due to loss of calcium and resulting in a porous condition of the bones; skeletal atrophy.

Ovaries The female sex glands (gonads) located on each side of the uterus that produce eggs and sex hormones, including oestrogen and progesterone as well as a smaller amount of androgens.

Palpitations Irregular or rapid heartbeats.

Parathyroid hormone A hormone secreted by the parathyroid glands that controls the body's calcium balance and metabolism.

Peak bone mass The ultimate or maximum amount of bone in the skeleton, usually achieved around the age of thirty years.

Pelvic floor muscles The muscles that form the anatomical 'floor' of the pelvic cavity and give support to the pelvic organs, including the uterus, bladder, and rectum.

Perimenopausal Referring to the years leading up to, during, and just after menopause (roughly ages forty to fifty-five).

Pharmacology The science of drugs and their chemical structures, uses, and beneficial and adverse effects.

Pituitary gland A mushroom-shaped gland that is connected by a stalk to the base of the brain. It manufactures many different hormones that in turn control other glands, such as the thyroid, the adrenal glands, and the ovaries.

Plethoric accumulations Congestion with blood.

Postmenopause The period of time after menopause.

Premenopause The period leading up to menopause. Generally four to five years long, it usually starts in the late forties, but it can begin any time after the age of thirty-five, and is characterized by hormonal imbalance.

Progesterone A sex hormone secreted by the corpus luteum of the ovary that acts to prepare the uterus for the possibility of pregnancy.

Progestogen A synthetic form of the hormone progesterone that is capable of producing menstrual bleeding.

Prolapse The abnormal dropping or protrusion of a bodily organ or structure, most often the rectum (bowel), bladder, uterus, or vagina.

Recommended daily allowance (RDA) The daily intake of various nutrients recommended by government health authorities. Consumption of the RDA of vitamins and minerals should guarantee an adequate amount of nutrients to avoid deficiency under normal circumstances. However, for optimal health, many nutritionists recommend consuming more than the RDA of certain nutrients, especially vitamin E, vitamin C, and beta-carotene.

Sex hormone binding globulin (SHBG) A protein in the blood that binds with and transports the sex hormones oestrogen, progesterone, and testosterone. When bound to SHBG, the sex hormones are inactive.

Stroke A condition in which the blood supply to the brain is disturbed to the extent that normal brain function is interrupted. A stroke may be mild and transitory, with no lasting effects, or it may cause permanent brain damage resulting in a degree of disability or even death.

Testosterone The primary sex hormone responsible for the development of masculine characteristics.

Thrombosis The formation of a blood clot in a blood vessel.

Tubal ligation A surgical sterilization procedure in which the fallopian tubes are cut and tied or pinched closed by the use of plastic rings or clips.

Uterus The female reproductive organ in which the fertilized egg implants and develops into a baby; the womb.

Vagina The genital cavity from the uterus to the vulva.

Vertebrae The bone segments that form the spinal column.

Vitamins A group of food factors essential for cellular metabolism and the maintenance of life.

Vulva The external female genitalia.

BIBLIOGRAPHY

Adlercreutz, H., Fotsis, T., et al, 'Determination of Urinary Lignans and Phytoestrogen Metabolites', *Journal of Steroid Biochemistry* 25 (5B) (November 1986): 791–7.

Armstrong, B.K., 'Oestrogen Therapy – Boon or Bane?' *Medical Journal of Australia* 148 (1988): 213–14.

Asch, R.H., and Greenblatt, R.B., 'Steroidogenesis in the Postmenopausal Ovary', *Clinics in Obstetrics and Gynaecology*, Vol. 4, No. 1 (April) 1977): 85–106.

Australian Menopause Society, 'Consensus Statement. Hormone Replacement Therapy and the Menopause', *Medical Journal of Australia* 155 (1991): 43–4.

Bergstrom, R., Falkeborn, M., Persson, I., et al. 'Hormone Replacement Therapy and the Risk of Stroke: Follow-up of a Population-based Cohort in Sweden', *Archives of Internal Medicine* 153 (10) (24 May 1993): 1201–9.

Buist, R., 'The Role of Nutrients in the Prevention of Heart Disease', Report to the seminar 'Nutrition in Disease Prevention', Sydney, Australia: Australian Council for Responsible Nutrition, 9 March 1992.

Cabot, Sandra, *The Body-Shaping Diet*, London: Boxtree, 1996.

Cordoza, Linda, et al. 'The Effects of Subcutaneous Hormone Implants During the Climacteric', *Maturitas* 5 (1984): 177–84.

Evans, Barbara, *Life Change*, London: Pan Books, 1979.

Gambrell, R.D., Jr, 'Oestrogen-Progestogen Replacement and Cancer Risk', *Hospital Practice* 15 (1990): 81–100.

Harrison, Lewis, *Making Fats and Oils Work for You*, Garden City Park, NY: Avery Publishing Group, 1990.

Henderson, Brian, 'An Epidemiological Evaluation of the Risks and Benefits of

HRT', *Proceedings of the Inaugural Scientific Meeting of the Australian Menopause Society*, Brisbane, Australia: Australian Menopause Society, September 1989.

Kaplan, F.S., 'Osteoporosis: Pathophysiology and Prevention', *Clinical Symposia*, Vol. 39 (1) Ciba-Geigy Corporation, 1987.

MacLennan, A.H., 'HRT Regimen for the Menopausal Woman', *Current Therapeutics*, March 1993: 43.

Rudman, Daniel, Feller, Axel, et al., 'Effects of Human Growth Hormone in Men Over 60 Years Old', *New England Journal of Medicine*, 323 (1) (5 July 1990): 1–6.

Setchell, K.D.R., Borriello, S.P., Hulme, P., Kirk, D.N., and Axelson, M., 'Nonsteroidal Estrogens of Dietary Origin: Possible Roles in Hormone-Dependent Disease', *American Journal of Clinical Nutrition* 40 (September 1984): 569–78.

Smith, R.W., Eyler, W.R., and Mellingen, R.C., 'On the Incidence of Senile Osteoporosis', *Annals of Internal Medicine* 52 (1960): 773–6.

Stampfer, M.J., Colditz, G.A., Willett, W.C., et al., 'Postmenopausal Estrogen Therapy and Cardiovascular Disease', *New England Journal of Medicine* 325 (11) (12 September 1991): 756–62.

Steinberg, K.K., Thacker, S.B., et al., 'A Meta-analysis of the Effect of Estrogen Replacement Therapy on the Risk of Breast Cancer', *Journal of the American Medical Association* 265 (1991): 1985–90.

Stevenson, J.C., Cust, M.P., Ganger, K.F., Hillard, T.C., Lees, B., and Whitehead, M.I., 'Effects of Transdermal Versus Oral Hormone Replacement Therapy on Bone Density in Spine and Proximal Femur in Postmenopausal Women', *Lancet* 336 No. II (1990): 265–9.

Studd, J.W., et al., 'Oestradiol and Testosterone Implants', *British Journal of Obstetrics and Gynaecology* 84 (1977): 314–15.

Tilyard, M.W., et al., 'Treatment of Postmenopausal Osteoporosis with Calcitriol or Calcium', *New England Journal of Medicine* 326 (1992): 357–62.

Watts, Nelson B., 'Intermittent Cyclical Etidronate Treatment of Postmenopausal Osteoporosis', *New England Journal of Medicine* 323 (12 July 1990): 73–9.

Weiss, N.S., Ure, C.L, Ballard, J.H., Williams, A.R., and Daling, J.R., 'Decreased Risk of Fractures of the Hip and Lower Forearm With Postmenopausal Use of Oestrogen', *New England Journal of Medicine* 303 (1980): 1195–8.

RESOURCE ORGANIZATIONS

Amarant Trust
Grant House
56-60 St John Street
London EC1M 4DT
0171 490 1644
Specialises in menopause therapy and counselling

British Homeopathic Association
27a Devonshire Street
London W1N 1RJ
0171 935 2163

British Society of Research on Aging
School of Biological Sciences
University of Manchester
3/239 Stopford Building
Oxford Road
Manchester M13 9PT
0161 275 5252

Continence Foundation
c/o The Dene Centre
Castle Farm Road
Newcastle-upon-Tyne NE3 1PH
0191 213 0050

The Endometriosis Society
35 Belgrave Square
London SW1X 8QB
0171 235 4137

General Council and Register of Osteopaths
56 London Street
Reading RG1 4SQ
01734 576585

Health Information Service
0800 66 55 44

Margaret Pyke Centre
15 Bateman's Buildings
Soho Square
London W1V 6JB
0171 734 9351
Offers assessment of suitability for HRT

Marie Stopes Centre
108 Whitfield Streer
London W1P 6BE
0171 388 2585
Call for local information; 50- minute 'Menocheck' offered to assess hormone levels

National Osteoporosis Society
PO Box 10
Radstock
Bath BA3 3YB
01761 432472

Women's Health Concern (WHC)
0181 780 3007 for details of regional counsellors

Women's Nutritional Advisory Service
PO Box 268
Lewes BN7 2QN
01273 487366
Ask also for details of telephone advice lines

INDEX

THE BODY-SHAPING DIET

How to order Dr Sandra Cabot's revolutionary *Body-Shaping Diet*

ORDER FORM

☐   I wish to order ☐☐ copy/copies of *The Body-Shaping Diet* including a complete weight-loss programme, tailor-made Body-Shaping Diet Plans and over 100 recipes, exercises and more @ £6.99 per copy.

Available at your local bookshop or direct from the publisher. Price and availability subject to change without notice.

Boxtree Cash Sales, PO Box 11, Falmouth, Cornwall, TR10 9EN

Please send cheque or postal order for the value of the book, and add the following for postage and packing:

UK including BFPO – £1.00 for one book, plus 50p for the second book, and 30p for each additional book ordered up to a £3.00 maximum.

OVERSEAS including Eire – £2.00 for the first book, plus £1.00 for the second book, and 50p for each additional book ordered.

OR please debit this amount from my ACCESS/VISA Card (delete as appropriate).

Card number ☐☐☐☐☐☐☐☐☐☐☐☐☐☐☐☐

Expiry date ☐☐/☐☐

Amount   £ . . . .

Signed   . . . .

Name   . . . .

Address   . . . .

. . . .

Post code   . . . .